BOOK TWO
the body makeover

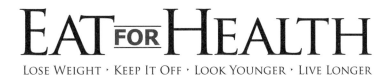

EAT FOR HEALTH

LOSE WEIGHT · KEEP IT OFF · LOOK YOUNGER · LIVE LONGER

BOOK TWO
the body makeover

EAT FOR HEALTH

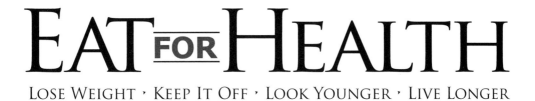

LOSE WEIGHT · KEEP IT OFF · LOOK YOUNGER · LIVE LONGER

Joel Fuhrman, M.D.

PUBLISHED BY

ϕϕ

Gift of Health Press

First Edition, Published March 2008

Contact:
Joel Fuhrman, MD
4 Walter Foran Boulevard, Suite 409
Flemington, NJ 08822

Printed in the United States
ISBN: 0-9799667-3-6

Library of Congress Control Number:
2007943877

Publishers Note:
Keep in mind that results vary from person to person. Some people have a medical history and/or condition that may warrant individual recommendations and in some cases drugs and even surgery. Do not start, stop or change medication without professional medical advice, and do not change your diet if you are ill or on medication except under the supervision of a competent physician. Neither this, nor any other book, is intended to take the place of personalized medical care or treatment.

A small percentage of the names used have requested their names be changed.

Book Design: Robyn Rolfes — Creative Syndicate, Inc.

TABLE OF CONTENTS

Change Your Health, Change Your Life

Book Two is the hands-on piece of your health makeover program. It is the practical step-by-step guide to menu planning, shopping and cooking that will allow you to implement the *Eat For Health* plan in your life. Continue to use Book One for re-reading and easy reference. Read Book Two in its entirety and then keep it in your kitchen for further reference to the menus and recipes. This book will take you through each phase of your transition as you step up to greater health. You will learn how to plan great menus and shop wisely for delicious, natural ingredients. Take some time during Phase One of this book to let me help you take inventory and set-up your kitchen. It is not enough to know what to do; you need to actually do it. Together, we will practice preparing recipes and eating healthful meals until they become a routine part of your lifestyle. As you progress, you will gradually replace your old way of eating.

The best way to fight the temptation to eat unhealthful, low-nutrient food is with two things: knowledge and great tasting meals. If you have the knowledge, but don't like what you are eating, you will ultimately fail. To make sure this doesn't happen, the recipes in Book Two are delicious, filled with many different ingredients and flavors to increase your enjoyment of eating. With these recipes and the knowledge you have gained, you will have the tools to ensure your success.

The only real hindrance to living healthier that you will still have to overcome is time. That is why planning your weekly menu to assure you have access to good-tasting, healthy food is crucial. Make sure you have easy-to-grab, nutritious food always available, wherever you go. When you become hungry and no healthy foods are around, you will be more likely to succumb to the temptation to eat something unhealthy. Why do you think "fast food" restaurants are so successful? They sell billions of burgers and fries because people don't want to take time and plan what they will be feeding themselves and their families. Americans are willing to sacrifice health and well-being for convenience. The irony is that a few hours of planning, shopping and cooking each week can secure long-term health and a more pleasurable and full life.

What good is living longer if we can't enjoy emotional and physical wellness and a full life? Applied to its fullest potential, high-nutrient eating can be the most effective therapy to reverse diabetes, high blood pressure and heart disease. It is the powerful medicine to get you well and keep you well in later life. Achieving good health through healthful living is your most important investment and it will pay you back with tremendous interest in your later years.

This book will make the commitment to that investment much easier. I have planned your menus in four separate levels, one for each phase of your health makeover. By the time you have completed Book Two, you will have established the menu-planning habit. Remember, there are good habits and bad habits. Unfortunately, bad habits are easily acquired and very tough to give up. Good habits may be more challenging to acquire and may take longer to develop, but they lead to a lifetime of good health. Work to develop the menu-planning habit so it is ingrained in you forever.

Try to move consecutively through the four phases of this program. If after you finish reading this book, you decide that you prefer to stay with any of the phases you may do so until you are ready to move forward. You may even choose to move back and forth or repeat the program. Any way you choose to use *Eat For Health* is fine. Eating from any of the phases is far healthier than eating the Standard American Diet and you will be rewarded accordingly.

Feel free to exchange any of the designated recipes for something else in the same phase or in a later phase. For example, it is fine to use a recipe from Phase Four while you are still in Phases One, Two or Three. There are recipes here for every meal, but in the real world, nobody needs to prepare all this food. Instead you can prepare enough of one dish so you can have leftovers for one, two, or even three subsequent days. The cooked foods and salad dressings and dips keep well and can be stored for up to four days. Phase One also contains some of my Quick and Easy Meal Suggestions for those days when you need shortcuts. You can also use healthy already prepared foods to speed up the food preparation process. At the back of this book is a list of recommended brands and product sources as well as spices and seasonings that can provide interesting flavors. (See Purchasing Guidelines, Page 90.)

Eat For Health allows you to gradually make the transition to great health as you adopt a nutritarian eating-style. However, for some people even the moderate changes in Phase One will be dramatic. The Phase One menus will show you how you can eat more high-nutrient foods than you are accustomed to, especially vegetables. As you become a nutritarian, you will see less of the foods you probably currently eat in large quantities, such as refined grains like pasta, cereal, and bread. You will add new things to your pantry and remove others. This portion of *Eat For Health* heavily utilizes the four "S"s: Smoothies, Soups, Salads and Sorbets. The tools you will learn here and all the others you have learned thus far will move you forward towards excellent health.

The Nutritional Rating System
Foods evaluated by my Nutritional Scoring System get two numbers: an ANDI Nutrient Score and a MANDI Point Value. ANDI stands for **Aggregate Nutrient Density Index**. These numbers are the scores that we listed and discussed in Chapter Three of Book One. The ANDI rating system scores foods on a scale of 0–1000. It is based on how many nutrients are in an equal caloric amount of each food. Using a specific calorie amount instead of weight or serving size is a more accurate way of obtaining a pure "nutrient per calorie" score, a reflection of the health equation. The most nutrient dense foods—green leafy vegetables such as kale, watercress and mustard greens—score 1000; all other foods are

then scored relative to them. We needed to use a scale of 0–1000 to give a true picture of the amazing nutrient density of vegetables compared to the foods that typically make up the Standard American Diet (SAD). Most SAD foods score less than 25.

MANDI stands for **Menu Aggregate Nutrient Density Index** and is much like the ANDI system, except if focuses on serving sizes instead of calories. The MANDI point system uses ANDI nutrient scores to assign point values to specific serving sizes of individual foods and recipes, allowing you to rate your daily menus. Using a simple equation, the ANDI, and the calories per serving, we calculate the MANDI and get a scoring system based on 100. A daily intake of 100 points of MANDI represents the ideal diet. The MANDI scores are another tool to help you live *Eat For Health* in your daily life, with foods and portion sizes that you typically encounter. Beginning on page 79, you will find point values for a variety of commonly eaten foods. If the serving size we have selected is different from what you are using, just divide or multiply accordingly. All of our recipes also have a MANDI nutrient point value as well as other nutrient information. For more details on how we calculate ANDI scores and MANDI points, see page 86.

Again, these scores are meant to help you in your quest for excellent health. They do not mean that you have to carry a calculator with you or be counting scores each time you eat. Over time, recognizing high-nutrient foods and dishes will become second nature to you and you will no longer need to calculate scores. You will be choosing high-nutrient foods and preparing high-nutrient meals automatically from what you have learned. In the beginning, it is helpful to approximate and add up your MANDI points to see your total point value for the day. You can use this to determine the nutrient density of your diet. Eating for superior health means you are attempting to eat as many points as possible. As you move from Phase One to Phase Four, the nutrient density of the menus I've planned here will increase gradually from adequate to superior.

The goal for Phase One is to reach a score of at least 60 for each day. The sample menus we provide show you how to put together meals that will give you an average score of 70 over the course of a week. You can use our menus or make up your own from the recipes we've given you, but still aim for at least 60 points each day. Since greens are highest in nutrient density, the key to getting a high score is to include as many greens in your diet as possible. Even though the Phase One menus are not the pinnacle of nutritional excellence, they still contain more than triple the level of nutrients consumed by most Americans. Sixty should be your minimum daily requirement, but to maximize disease reversal and longevity you can do even better. That is why we have four phases, to get you gradually up to eating a diet that earns 80, 90 or even 100 nutrient points. The scores were designed to make 100 the ideal score, but it will be easier for a male eating more calories to reach this total and harder for women consuming fewer calories. Don't overeat to try to pump up the total. Try to get as high a score as you can without snacking or overeating. It is best to stop eating before you feel full or stuffed. As you modify your eating-style to move up to a higher level of nutritional excellence you will be able to maximize the body's miraculous self-healing properties and slow the process of aging.

Four Levels of Nutritional Excellence
In Phase One, you will learn to eliminate fried foods and make substitutions for low-nutrient foods, such as ice cream, chips, candy, and white flour products. You will also eliminate foods like cheese and butter that are high in saturated fats, and your cooking techniques will use a minimal amount of oil. Salt is also significantly reduced. The foods and recipes are designed to taste good without salt; nevertheless, allow time for your taste buds to regain their sensitivity to salt. After the first month of not using salt you will be amazed at how much more flavor you can taste in an unsalted dish.

Phase Two includes only five servings of animal products per week and we continue to reduce grains to allow vegetables to be an even larger portion of your total caloric intake. When you incorporate more and more nutrient-rich produce in your diet, you automatically increase your intake of plant fibers, lignins, and plant sterols, and lower the glycemic index of your diet and the level of saturated fat, salt and other negative elements without having to think about it. Your ability to appreciate natural flavors will improve because you are losing your dependence on salt and sugar. More beans and nuts are added to your diet to replace animal products. It will become obvious that eating for great health has little to do with portion control and much more to do with content control.

Your nutrition makeover will be well underway by the time you arrive at Phase Three. More unhealthy foods are eliminated, sodium levels continue to decrease, and your diet becomes even more nutrient rich. You will learn how to make great tasting healthy salad dressings and dips from nuts and nut butters, instead of oil. My creative recipes will ensure that you don't miss your old eating style. As you move up to Phase Three and have more experience, you will become skilled at rapidly estimating the nutrient points in foods, recipes, and menus. You will instinctively know how much high-nutrient food you need to eat each day and you may not have to count anymore. Your brain will automatically direct you to collect nutrient points as you make your daily food choices. You will learn, practice, and eventually master the technique until it is effortless.

Arrival at Phase Four means you are ready to reach for the nutritional pinnacle of excellence! At this level, we make every calorie count. Animal products are reduced to two servings per week. The final cooking technique to master is the art of making green smoothies, also called blended salads. Here you are at peak nutrient density.

Nutrition without Points
I am often asked if you can *eat for health* past Phase One without counting MANDI points, and the answer is yes. If you do not want to worry about counting points, below are the main things you should concentrate on to assure you are eating a high-nutrient diet that at least reaches the Phase One recommended level.

1. Eat a large raw salad each day. The amount of leafy lettuce and other leafy greens such as spinach and arugula in the salad should amount to at least 5 ounces. Double this quantity of leafy greens if you want to jump up to a higher level of excellence.

2. Add other raw vegetables (besides the leafy greens) such as tomatoes, shredded carrots, cabbage, beets, snow peas, or raw broccoli to the salad so the total of raw vegetables for the day amounts to at least 12 ounces of food.

3. Consume a double-portion serving of steamed green vegetables (at least 12 ounces a day). Vegetables such as asparagus, artichokes, kale, collards, broccoli, Brussels sprouts, string beans, baby bok choy, and others should be eaten every day. You can also do this by adding these greens to a soup.

4. Eat ½ cup to one cup of beans daily in a vegetable soup, on your salad, as an ingredient to a main dish or in a dip.

5. Eat at least one ounce of raw seeds or nuts daily, preferably in one of the delicious salad dressings or dips you can find within this book. Try to use more seeds and less nuts.

6. Eat at least four fresh fruits daily. Try to eat some berries, cherries or other high-nutrient fruits regularly.

7. Have some fresh squeezed vegetable juice either by itself or part of your soup base on most days.

8. Measure and control the type and amount of animal products consumed. Do not eat more than one serving of animal products a day and limit the size of the portion so it is under five ounces. That means no larger than the size of a deck of cards. Then as you move forward and learn the recipes here try to move up to the next phase of nutritional excellence by reducing animal products further. It would be a significant health achievement if you do not have more than one serving of animal products every other day. In other words, whether you have two eggs, chicken in your salad or soup, or a turkey sandwich on whole grain pita, make the next day a strict vegetarian day. Keep full-fat dairy very limited and do not eat processed or salted meats.

9. Reduce and measure your salt intake. Do not cook with salt in the home. The goal is to learn many of my delicious recipes featured here that are flavorful without salt and learn how to cook without it. Do not eat soup or sauces in restaurants; they are too high in sodium. Always order the dressing on the side and ask if the food can be prepared without the sauce. If you are using a packaged or third-party prepared food, make sure the

sodium content is not more than 400 mg, and make sure that this is the only sodium-extra food that you consume that day. In other words, limit your salt consumption to 400 mg per day in addition to the natural sodium found in all the unsalted produce and other dishes you eat each day.

10. Get most of your starch intake from carrots, peas, sweet potato, squash and beans, not from flour products and white potato. Do not eat white flour products. If you're using bread and pasta, use limited amounts, not more than one serving per day and, of course, make sure it is 100 percent whole grain.

11. Limit your consumption of oil to one tablespoon daily. Oil is a fattening, low-nutrient food. If you eat something cooked with oil, make sure you do not use oil on your salad that day.

12. Use the nutrient density chart on the next page to help you focus your food consumption so you eat larger amounts of raw and cooked vegetables and fresh fruit and less animal products, baked goods, oils and prepared sweets.

Whether using the MANDI points or not, as you progress through the four phases of this book, keep the nutrient density chart in your mind. You can even keep it out for an easy, visual reminder of your goals.

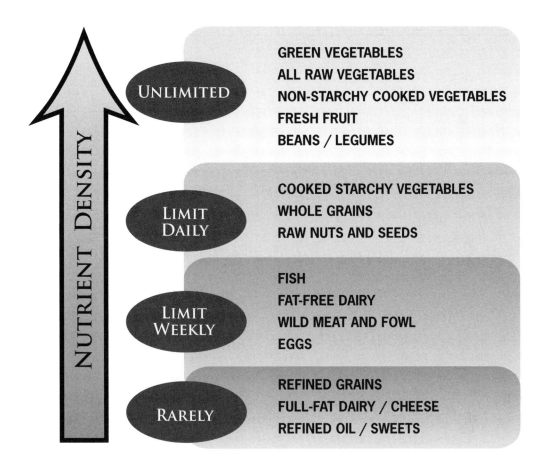

Take your time going through the eating phases in order. If possible try all of the recipes and pick out the ones you like the best. The phases have been designed to change your food preferences as you move through them.

OVERVIEW OF THE FOUR PHASES

	PHASE ONE
MANDI	60
ANIMAL PRODUCTS	8 servings/week
SODIUM*	1600 mg/day
GRAINS**AND STARCHY VEGETABLE***	14/week
FATS/OILS	1 Tbsp of olive oil or replaceable substitute**** per day
BEVERAGE	Water, fresh squeezed juice, herbal teas. If desired 1 cup coffee/tea
COOKING METHODS	Reducing salt and substituting other seasonings — Cooking with minimal oil — Creating fruit smoothies — Water sautéing
CONCEPTS	Reducing sodium — Increasing fruit and green vegetables

*The amount of sodium allotted includes that which is naturally occurring in foods (approximately 700mg) plus what is added.
**Only use whole grains: bread, tortillas, cooked and dry cereals, pasta, and brown rice.

PHASE TWO	PHASE THREE	PHASE FOUR
75	90	100+
5 servings/week	3 servings/week	2 servings/week
1200 mg/day	1000 mg/day	900 mg/day
12/week	10/week	7/week
1 Tbsp of olive oil or replaceable substitute**** per day	2 Tbsp of olive oil per week	Minimal
Water, fresh squeezed juice, herbal tea. If desired 1 cup coffee/tea	Water, fresh squeezed juice, herbal tea.	Water, fresh squeezed juice, and vegetable juices
Soups and stews	Salad dressings- Using nuts, seeds, avocados and tahini in place of oil — Sweetening nutrient dense desserts with dates and dried fruit	Juicing and vegetable smoothies (blended salads)
Adding more beans and nuts — Reducing animal products — Continuing to reduce sodium — Adding more green vegetables	Eliminating oil and caffeine — Continuing to reduce animal products and sodium — Adding more green vegetables and fruit	Maximizing nutrient density and absorption

***Starchy vegetables include: corn, white potatoes, sweet potatoes, squash, carrots, and parsnips.
****Substitutes include: non-dairy spreads without trans-fats and hydrogenated oil such as Earth Balance, Smart Balance, and Spectrum.

Changing your body for the better is an exciting journey and a rewarding accomplishment. This will be a process that requires time and effort and the ability to learn from mistakes. Give your taste buds time to adjust to new food choices. Be easy on yourself if you slip up, but don't give up the plan. Get right back on track quickly. The only failure is to stop trying. You will experience more rewards from this program as you stick to it longer. As you increase nutrients in your diet, your desire for unhealthy food will gradually diminish. You will reap the rewards of superior health, mental clarity, youthful vigor, and ideal weight proportionally to the effort you put into this program.

Try Not to Snack
For maximum success, it is best to eat only when you are hungry and to stop eating when you feel satisfied. This will require less willpower as you start to satisfy your body's nutritional and volume requirements. During Phase One, I want you to try to get back in touch with your body's signals. Try to eat only when you feel hungry and as time progresses, pay attention to see if you can develop the ability to distinguish true hunger—felt in the throat—from the symptoms of toxic hunger. Remember, the symptoms of toxic hunger, which are caused by withdrawal, won't turn off until you have provided your body with adequate nutrients and your body has had time to build up a nutrient reserve in its tissues. This could take a few weeks to a few months, so be patient.

Eating when hungry usually translates into a three meal-per-day format, without snacking. Unless you are a dedicated athlete or a physical laborer, you probably don't burn enough calories to justify snacking. Snacking is most often recreational eating, without true hunger present. It has negative effects, including the following.

1) Snacking usually results in the consumption of a higher amount of calories each week.

2) Snacking means you will not experience true hunger before meals, thus diminishing enjoyment of food.

3) In animal studies, eating less frequently results in increased lifespan.

4) The digestive tract needs adequate rest to build up digestive enzymes for proper digestion.

5) Detoxification and cellular repair occur more efficiently when the body is not digesting.

6) The healthier you eat, the faster you will diminish the desire to eat between meals and the symptoms of toxic hunger.

Some helpful hints to combat snacking are:

- Eat a salad or raw vegetables with a dip to start both lunch and dinner.

- Keep lots of frozen fruits and vegetables and pre-washed fresh items in your home.

- Have cooked greens or soups with greens at every lunch and dinner.

- Don't eat after 8:00 p.m.

- Have a fruit sorbet or fruit desert after dinner and then clean the kitchen, clean your teeth, and end eating for the day.

Eliminate Temptation

It is best if you can get rid of all the unhealthy food in your kitchen. If it's not in the house, you won't have to fight unnecessary temptation and you will not be faced with the constant decision of whether or not to eat it. Instead, stock up on nutrient-rich, healthy foods. This strategy can be one of the most important steps toward healthful living. Eventually, healthy food can taste just as good as unhealthy options, you just have to learn the best ways to prepare it and how to get your taste buds in shape to enjoy it.

If your family does not want to join your health makeover, then create a separate area in the pantry and refrigerator for your foods. It is more challenging if you have to make unhealthy foods for your family while you're in the midst of your own health makeover, but let no obstacles stop you. Remember, by making yourself healthier and enjoying it, you are opening the door for others to potentially follow your lead. Share what you are learning and your excitement about your changes, and let each person come to their own conclusions in their own time. It is very likely that when your family and friends see you looking and feeling better, they will want to know more about what you are doing, and you will eventually have others join you on your quest for better health.

Shopping

This healthy makeover will require some brushing up on your shopping skills. In Phase One of this book we will take some time to learn how to shop for high-nutrient foods, which are mostly in the produce aisle. Since it is necessary to consume a variety of fresh fruits and vegetables, I recommend that you shop twice a week. You will use the main shopping trip of the week to stock up on staples and produce for three or four days. Your second trip of the week can be a short trip to restock fresh fruits and vegetables. You will spend most of your time in the produce, health food, and frozen foods sections. The supermarket can be filled with temptation at the beginning of your health transformation, so try to avoid certain aisles. The center aisles of most stores contain the most heavily processed foods, so consider them non-existent. What you don't see can't tempt you!

Reading Food Labels

The most important point about food labels is that you should avoid foods that have labels. Unless it is a frozen fruit or vegetable, if it comes in a box, bag, or jar, it is likely processed and contains an insignificant amount of nutrients per calorie. The goal is to rarely look at a food label and rarely buy a food that has a label. When you do look at a label, be selective and use good judgment. Food labels contain some information to guide you about the healthfulness of a product if you know what to look for and how to interpret it, but the packaging of a food product tells you little, if anything at all, about the nutritional content of the food. The manufacturer designs the packaging based on what they think will attract the consumer and ultimately sell their product.

The ingredient list is the most important bit of information on the package. It is often difficult to find and in very small print. Most people don't bother to take the time to look for it or read it. This is where you will find out what's really in a product and how healthy or unhealthy it is. Inspect labels before you add an item to your shopping cart! Reading labels will mostly reinforce the idea that you should put the food back on the shelf. You want to avoid foods whose first few ingredients contain white flour (called wheat flour) and any type of sweetener, such as corn syrup. Ingredients are listed on the label according to quantity, in descending order based on weight (from most to least). As a general rule of thumb, if the list of ingredients is long and you cannot pronounce most of them, there are probably a lot of chemical additives in the product, and you're risking your health by eating it.

Be sure to read the ingredients even when purchasing foods from a health food store or when the rest of the packaging is trying to convince you the food is healthy. For example, watch out for statements like these on packages:

- NATURAL FRUIT FLAVORS

- WITH REAL FRUIT JUICE

- ALL NATURAL INGREDIENTS

- NO ARTIFICIAL PRESERVATIVES

- 100% NATURAL

- REAL FRUIT

- NO PRESERVATIVES

- NO ARTIFICIAL INGREDIENTS

Statements like these do not mean there are no harmful additives in the product or that the products are healthful, they simply mean the manufacturer hopes you'll think there are no harmful ingredients. For example, the ingredients list from a loaf of bread that states on the label, 'ALL NATURAL INGRE-DIENTS,' and 'NO ARTIFICIAL PRESERVATIVES ADDED,' reads as follows:

Enriched wheat flour (wheat flour, malted barley, niacin, reduced iron, thiamine mononitrate, riboflavin), water, high fructose corn syrup, yeast, wheat bran, vital wheat gluten, butter. Contains 2% or less of each of the following: rye meal, corn flour, molasses, rolled whole wheat, salt, dough conditioners (ammonium sulfate, sodium stearoyl lactylate), brown sugar, honey, vinegar, oatmeal, soy flour, mono and diglycerides, partially hydrogenated soybean oil.

As we take a look at this list, we see the first two ingredients listed are white flour and sugar. It is junk food.

- Enriched wheat flour is white flour. The bran and the germ portion of the whole wheat, which are rich in vitamins and minerals, have been refined out. To compensate for refining out approximately 20 nutrients, they add back four. Use only whole wheat flour, it must have the word whole on the label.

- High fructose corn syrup is a concentrated form of sugar derived from corn.

- Dough conditioners, in general, can cause mineral deficiencies, and ammonium sulfate in particular may cause mouth ulcers, nausea, and kidney and liver problems.

- Brown sugar is merely white sugar with molasses added.

- Partially hydrogenated soybean oil is a trans fat associated with heart disease, breast and colon cancer, atherosclerosis and elevated cholesterol. It is even worse than saturated fat.

As you can see, this "all-natural" bread will not help you on your road to health. Even if you didn't know the particular detriments of each ingredient, taking the time to read that it's main ingredients are white flour and sugar, and that the rest of the list is lengthy, would tell you to leave it on the shelf.

When looking at labels, we also need to be aware of sodium levels. A lot of sodium is "hidden" in processed foods from spaghetti sauce to canned soup to frozen dinners. Obviously, if you see the word "salt" on a food label, you know salt is in the product. But baking soda and Monosodium glutamate (MSG) contain sodium, too. To avoid excess sodium, try to avoid products with: brine, disodium phosphate, garlic salt, onion salt, sodium alginate, sodium benzoate, sodium caseinate, sodium citrate, sodium hydroxide, sodium nitrate, sodium pectinate, sodium proprionate, and sodium sulfite. Also avoid anything using the words "pickled," "cured," "broth," and "soy sauce." They all indicate high sodium. Just because a product says that it has reduced sodium or is light in sodium, it does not mean it is a low-salt product. It only means it has less than the higher-salt version of the product. Lots of these products still contain much too much salt for good health.

IF THE LABEL SAYS...	IT MEANS...
Sodium free/salt free	Less than 5 mg sodium added per serving
Very low sodium	Less than 35 mg sodium added per serving
Low sodium	Less than 140 mg sodium per serving
Reduced sodium	At least 25% less sodium than the original product
Light in sodium	At least 50% less sodium than the original product
Unsalted / No added salt	No salt added during processing (not necessarily sodium-free)

In addition to sodium, most processed foods contain a litany of food additives with toxic properties. Substances such as artificial colors, sweeteners, stabilizers, nitrates, and preservatives are often linked to cancer in lab animals and may be harmful or cancer promoting in humans. They are best avoided. You can find out what additives are in a given food by knowing how to read the label.

Lets take a look at a sample food label to discover what else we can learn from this packaging.

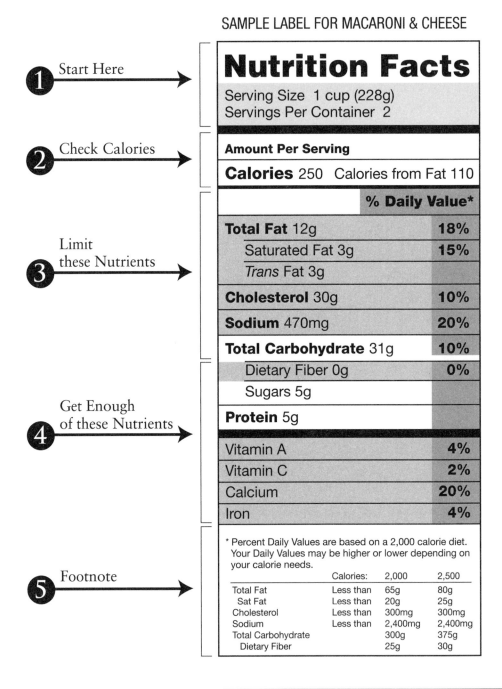

SAMPLE LABEL FOR MACARONI & CHEESE

① Start Here

② Check Calories

③ Limit these Nutrients

④ Get Enough of these Nutrients

⑤ Footnote

Nutrition Facts

Serving Size 1 cup (228g)
Servings Per Container 2

Amount Per Serving

Calories 250   Calories from Fat 110

	% Daily Value*
Total Fat 12g	**18%**
Saturated Fat 3g	**15%**
Trans Fat 3g	
Cholesterol 30g	**10%**
Sodium 470mg	**20%**
Total Carbohydrate 31g	**10%**
Dietary Fiber 0g	**0%**
Sugars 5g	
Protein 5g	
Vitamin A	**4%**
Vitamin C	**2%**
Calcium	**20%**
Iron	**4%**

* Percent Daily Values are based on a 2,000 calorie diet. Your Daily Values may be higher or lower depending on your calorie needs.

	Calories:	2,000	2,500
Total Fat	Less than	65g	80g
Sat Fat	Less than	20g	25g
Cholesterol	Less than	300mg	300mg
Sodium	Less than	2,400mg	2,400mg
Total Carbohydrate		300g	375g
Dietary Fiber		25g	30g

The Serving Size

Serving Size 1 cup (228g)
Servings Per Container 2

The first place to start when you look at the Nutrition Facts label is the serving size and the number of servings in the package. Serving sizes are standardized to make it easier to compare similar foods; they are provided in familiar units, such as cups or pieces, followed by the metric amount, e.g., the number of grams. The size of the serving on the food package influences the number of calories and the nutrient amounts listed on the top part of the label. Pay attention to the serving size, especially how many servings there are in the food package. The amount specified by the manufacturer as a serving size might not be what you or any other consumer typically eats in a serving. The manufacturer may have stated an extremely low serving size to camouflage the high level of trans fat or sodium in the product.

 Calories
(and Calories from Fat)

Amount Per Serving

Calories 250   Calories from Fat 110

Remember, the main focus of the *Eat For Health* program is not the number of calories, but the quality of calories. It is the amount of nutrients per calorie that determines the quality of the calories. Eating low-nutrient calories is not only linked to being overweight and becoming diabetic, but it is also a chief cause of heart disease and cancer.

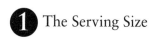

Total Fat 12g	**18%**
Saturated Fat 3g	**15%**
Trans Fat 3g	
Cholesterol 30g	**10%**
Sodium 470mg	**20%**

The nutrients listed first are the ones Americans generally eat in excess amounts. Eating processed food can give us extra saturated fat, cholesterol, and sodium, but a serious problem in processed food can also be the trans fat or hydrogenated oils. Ignore the percentage recommendations because they are overly permissive. Eating according to those can take 20 or 30 years off your life from a heart attack or a stroke. Avoid processed foods that are high in sodium, meaning they contain over 300 mg of sodium per serving.

Dietary Fiber 0g	0%

Vitamin A	4%
Vitamin C	2%
Calcium	20%
Iron	4%

Most Americans don't get enough dietary fiber, vitamins, and minerals from their diet. You might want to look for foods that contain more of the nutrients on the label, but because the list of nutrients is so narrow, it's not really helpful. When you focus on only a few nutrients, it can make a food look satisfactory when it actually contains a very narrow complement of nutrients. The little bit of nutrients in or added to processed foods can be confusing. For example, Cocoa Puffs and Fruit Loops have some nutrients added to them to make their labels look better, but these are not healthy foods. The range of nutrients added back to these and other processed foods is too narrow and the level of phytochemicals is too low. Natural foods not only contain larger amounts of these basic nutrients, but also contain thousands of phytochemicals that have never even been named. Since this short list of nutrients that manufacturers provide is not helpful, it makes sense to ignore it.

Quick Guide to Reading Labels:
- Food labels list ingredients in descending order. What's first on the ingredient list is present in the highest quantity.

- Do not purchase foods that contain flour or sweeteners in the first four ingredients or that contain any hydrogenated (trans) fat, or chemical additives.

- Avoid foods that have more then 300 mg sodium per serving.

Navigating the Food Categories

1) VEGETABLES

Since vegetables and fruit contain the most nutrients, the first part of your health makeover is to include more of them in your menus. Let's go over how you can do this.

The first thing to include in your daily menu is a salad, either at lunch or dinner. Eating raw vegetables every day is an important part of a healthy diet. A large head of romaine weighs about 1 pound, while a bagged salad mix has the ounces marked and is usually four to five ounces. For two people, I often mix a one-pound head of lettuce with a bag of mixed baby greens. If you feel the serving of raw vegetables is too much for you, only eat what feels comfortable. Don't force yourself to eat more, but I do want you to think of the **salad as the main dish** and eat as many raw greens and other raw vegetables as you can. Use any assortment of chopped or shredded raw vegetables. Health food stores often have sprouted lentils and beans, which are nice additions to any salad. You can also easily sprout grains and seeds yourself. Try adding new things to your salad like frozen peas and corn, very finely chopped onion, canned beans, snow pea pods, leftover cooked potato or sweet potato, leftover steamed vegetables, and fresh or dried fruits.

The most critical mistake to avoid in salads is adding too many calories from oil or too much salt from a commercial salad dressing. At 120 calories a tablespoon, oil calories can add up fast. Try many of the delicious, healthy dressing and dip suggestions in this book or use a low-calorie, low-salt dressing. I often whip up a quick salad dressing/dip by blending some leftover soup with a small handful of raw cashews and some nutritional yeast. (See my Purchasing Guidelines on page 90 for brands that will help you avoid dressing pitfalls.)

Stock your pantry with raw vegetables and eat as much as you can of these, either raw or steamed, and with the delicious dressings or dips contained in this book. Most vegetables are so low in calories and so nutrient rich that even if you eat large amounts you will not gain weight, and if you are overweight, eating more of these will help you lose excess pounds.

VEGETABLES TO EAT RAW

Celery	Daikon Radish	All varieties of leafy greens
Zucchini	Cauliflower	
Snow Peas	Radishes	Cucumber
Carrots	Asparagus	Green Beans
Summer Squash	Sprouts	Endive Leaves
Broccoli	Fennel	Bell Peppers
Tomatoes	Baby Bok Choy	Sugar Snap Peas

The non-starchy, low-calorie vegetables we often eat cooked include green vegetables such as string beans, broccoli, artichokes, asparagus, zucchini, kale, collards, cabbage, Brussels sprouts, bok choy, okra, Swiss chard, turnip greens and escarole, as well as the non-green, low-starch, low calorie vegetables such as eggplant, peppers, tomatoes, mushrooms, onion, garlic, hearts of palm, cauliflower, spaghetti squash, and water chestnuts.

LOW-STARCH, LOW-CALORIE VEGETABLES THAT ARE NOT GREEN

eggplant	mushrooms	spaghetti squash
garlic	onions	tomatoes
hearts of palm	colorful peppers	waterchestnuts

If you are someone who needs to lose weight, the secret is to eat more of the raw vegetables, green vegetables and low-starch, low-calorie vegetables above. The more of these high-nutrient, low-calorie foods you eat, the easier it will be to lose weight. The recipes for lightly steamed vegetables, vegetable stews, vegetable soups, and vegetable main courses that follow in these pages will have you increasing these high-nutrient vegetables as you progress through each phase.

Frozen vegetables are also a convenient option. They are picked ripe and flash-frozen right on the farm, so they are rich in micronutrients. Feel free to substitute frozen vegetables in any of the recipes. Canned vegetables are water-logged and not as nutritious.

Starchy vegetables include winter squashes, corn, potatoes, cooked carrots, sweet potatoes, yams and pumpkins. Since they are more calorically dense than the non-starchy vegetables, they are limited to one serving daily for those who need to lose weight. It is convenient to place whole grains, such as brown and wild rice, quinoa, millet, and whole wheat in this category too, but keep in mind that the colorful, high-starch vegetables such as carrots and sweet potato are higher in nutrients compared to the grains.

2) Nuts, Seeds, and Avocado

High-fat plant foods are high in the essential fatty acids that your body needs. Even though these foods are higher in calories and fats, their use is linked to lower risk of heart attacks and strokes. Keep lots of raw nuts, seeds, flaxseed, and avocados on hand because they are your preferred fatty food and should be used in salad dressings and other recipes. These foods are higher in calories, so if you are trying to lose weight it is helpful not to use more than half an avocado per day and limit the quantity of seeds and nuts to a one ounce serving per day for a female and less than two ounces (1/4 cup) a day for a male. For those of you who are thin and want to gain weight or need more calories to fuel your high athletic efforts, more of these higher-fat, higher-calorie nuts and seeds can be used in your diet to meet your higher caloric needs. I also recommend pregnant women consume at least 2 ounces of seeds and nuts a day. Nuts and seeds are about 175 calories an ounce.

3) FRUITS

You should always keep a good supply of fresh fruit on hand. It is the ultimate "convenience" food. Try to eat a variety of fruits: apples, apricots, bananas, blueberries, cherries, clementines, dates, figs, grapefruit, grapes, kiwis, kumquats, mangoes, melons, nectarines, oranges, papayas, peaches, pears, persimmons, pineapples, plums, pomegranates, raspberries, strawberries, and tangerines. Try some exotic fruits to add variety and interest to your diet.

If you are diabetic or on an aggressive weight loss plan, eat more fruits that are lower in sugar such as berries, green or Granny Smith apples, melons, grapefruit, oranges, kiwis and papaya and less of the higher calorie fruits such as mangos, grapes, bananas, pineapple and peaches. Fruit does not need to be avoided if diabetic, just limited to two fresh fruits with breakfast and one with lunch and dinner. Those with diabetes should exclude fruit juice and not use much dried fruit.

Frozen fruit can be a convenient substitute when fresh isn't available. The nutritional value is comparable to fresh, but like vegetables, avoid the canned variety because they are not as nutritious, they often have sweeteners added, and they have already lost most water-soluble nutrients.

4) BEANS OR LEGUMES

Stock up on dried and canned beans. These plant foods will help you feel full and curb your desire for sweets. Most of our soup and stew recipes also contain legumes. Canned beans are convenient and easy to add to a salad to make a filling meal. The unsalted canned beans that are available in health food stores or the health food section of your supermarket are preferable. If using salted canned beans, rinse them before using. Dried legumes and beans are a very economical, high-nutrient food. If you are on a food budget, use lots of dried beans in your cooking and also sprout whole beans and grains for some of your vegetable needs. You can soak the whole beans in water overnight in a jar and rinse and drain the water out for the next few days, until you have the sprouts to use.

If beans give you gas or bloating, it helps if you make sure you chew them very well. It takes some time for your digestive tract to learn how to digest them better, so you may have to start out with a smaller quantity and increase the amount gradually. Don't stop eating beans entirely. It will make things worse when you try to eat them again. Instead, just eat a smaller amount every day.

5) WHOLE GRAINS

Whole grains include barley, buckwheat (kasha), millet, oats, quinoa, brown rice and wild rice, all of which are high in fiber. Just because a food is called "whole grain" you can't assume it is a good food. Many whole grain cold cereals are so processed that they do not have a significant fiber per serving ratio and have lost most of their nutritional value. The more coarsely ground grains are absorbed into the bloodstream more slowly and therefore curtail appetite better.

Whole grain hot cereals are less processed than cold cereals and come up with better nutritional scores. They can be soaked in water overnight so you do not have to cook them in the morning. For example, if you throw some rolled oats in a covered container with raisins and water, it will be soft and ready to eat the next morning, either cold or quickly warmed. Some recommended hot whole grain cereals are non-instant oatmeal, Roman Meal, Steel Cut Oats, Wheatena, Ralston High Fiber and Quaker Multigrain.

6) ANIMAL PRODUCTS

As you move through this program the goal is to limit animal products to ten percent of caloric intake or less. On the days when you do include animal products in your menu, try to keep the serving size less than five ounces.

Phase One of this book permits more animal products than I generally recommend. It still is a large reduction in animal product intake for most people and an important first step. If you are comfortable eating less animal products in Phase One, go for it. Full-fat dairy, such as cheese and butter, are the foods with the highest saturated fat content, so choose mostly from fat-free dairy products, and for the same reason, try to choose white meat fowl, fish and eggs. Avoid processed meats, barbecued meats, luncheon meats, bacon, hot dogs, and any pickled, darkened, blackened, barbecued or over-cooked animal products. They contain high levels of cancer-promoting substances called carcinogens.

Eating in Restaurants

Dining out can be challenging when transitioning to a healthy diet. The first step when going out to eat is trying to find a restaurant that will have some healthful options. Many restaurants will cater to your needs and preferences. Call ahead and ask. Eat early before the restaurant gets very crowded so the staff will have time to modify a dish or make something for you.

If your restaurant meal is a breakfast, stay away from the bread, bagels, and breakfast sweets. It is easy to find oatmeal and fruit or eggs. For lunch and dinner, ask for an extra side of steamed vegetables instead of pasta or white rice to accompany your main dish. Patronize restaurants that have salad bars to get your money's worth. You can also order Asian vegetable dishes that are steamed or water sauteed with the dressing or sauce on the side. Because soups are made in advance in restaurants and are always very high in salt, it is best that you do not eat soups out. Stick with salads and a main dish. I often order a double-sized salad and let them charge me double. Ask the waiter not to bring bread to the table, so you are not tempted to fill up before the meal. Always order the salad dressing on the side so you can use their high-salt dressings sparingly. You can also ask if they have olive oil to use instead of butter on bread or potato or to use (with or without vinegar) instead of the high-salt salad dressing.

Helpful Tools

Your journey to excellent health will be made much easier if you have all of the tools you need in your kitchen. You may already have everything you need to start cooking, but take a few minutes to make sure you are supplied with these important basics:

- Colander

- Garlic press

- Food chopper

- Vegetable juicer

- High-powered blender

- Pressure cooker

A powerful blender such as the Vita-Mix is very helpful. Only the more expensive, high-powered blenders will be able to make fruit sorbets from frozen fruits and creamy dressings and dips from nuts and seeds. They can also blend vegetables effortlessly for your fruit or green smoothies. It is a good investment that will last a lifetime. Cooking soups and stews with a pressure cooker is helpful because it produces healthy and tasty food fast. You can prepare a soup or bean dish in less than half the time.

CONSIDERING CALORIES:

Try to let hunger be your guide to determine the right amount of calories. If you eat when you are truly hungry and do not eat when you are not, you will not over-consume calories. Strive for the most micronutrients you can muster with fewer calories than you would normally consume. Ideally, this eating-style should make you feel comfortable eating the amount of calories that will automatically and naturally bring you to, and eventually sustain you at, your ideal weight. Certainly, I do not want you to strive for a higher MANDI score by overeating. In fact, a high nutrient density diet is the foundation needed to comfortably desire fewer calories, so the calories desired match the calories required to maintain one's ideal weight and maximize your health. Achieving hunger before meals enhances taste and eating pleasure, so eating the appropriate number of calories also makes eating more enjoyable. Adjust the amount you eat, so that you are hungry again before the next meal. If you are not hungry at mealtime, you likely overate at the previous meal and you need to adjust your caloric intake accordingly so this does not happen regularly. You some-times may have to delay eating, or even skip a meal, so that you only eat when you are hungry.

Keep in mind, that even though the calories in the following menus may contain 1800 – 2000 calories, some people will require less and some people more. The average woman in America consumes about 1600. So if you are female, and do not exercise frequently, these menus may contain too many calories for you. You can easily reduce the calories by eating less or by reducing some of the nuts/seeds and dried fruits in the recipes. If you are a highly active male, you may need to increase the calories by eating more food or by using more of the higher calorie nuts/seeds in the menus or recipes.

Generally, you should always try to maximize the nutrient value of what you eat and, as you progress through the phases, aim for a diet-style that provides about 100 MANDI points per 2000 calories or about 50 points per 1000 calories. The MANDI score is a guide to help you measure the nutritional quality of your diet and to steer you toward higher nutrient levels with less calories.

COOKING FOR PHASE ONE

The delicious recipes in Phase One begin to put the spotlight on nutrient-rich fruits and vegetables. Compared to the standard diet, animal products start to take a back seat. This may be an opportunity for you to explore some new vegetables, beans, and grains. Braised Bok Choy, which is paired with a Spiced Tilapia, is a simple, nutrient-dense recipe that may expose you to new flavors. At the start, you will be eating less red meat and cheese and the animal products you do eat will be lower in fat. You will find that interesting new flavors replace salt and sugar.

Low- or no-salt versions of canned beans, canned tomato products and other ingredients are specified. (See my Purchasing Guidelines, page 90.) This may require exploring the health food aisle of your supermarket or a health food store. When recipes like the Pasta with Roasted Vegetables use olive oil for cooking, only a small amount of oil is needed.

The Fast Black Bean Soup on Day Three is an easy and delicious introduction to high-nutrient soup making. Low-sodium prepared canned soup and frozen vegetables are used to reduce cooking time. Carrot juice is often used as a soup ingredient. Bottled carrot juice can be purchased from a health food store for convenience, but you really cannot compare the flavor of the soup when you use carrot juice made fresh from organic carrots. Some health food stores have juice bars where you could purchase fresh squeezed juices for use in your soups if you do not want to juice carrots at home. For those busy days, take a look at the Quick and Easy Meal Suggestions we have included after the Phase 1 sample menus.

The first basic cooking technique you will learn is water sautéing (also called sweating). This is used instead of cooking with oil. Water sautéing is simple and great for stir-fries, sauces and many other dishes. To water sauté, heat a skillet on high heat until water sputters when dropped on the pan. Use small amounts of water in the hot skillet, wok, or pan, covering occasionally and adding more water when necessary until vegetables are tender.

NUTRITIONAL COMPARISON

SAD MENU vs. *EAT FOR HEALTH* PHASE ONE MENU

SAD SAMPLE MENU	MANDI POINTS	EAT FOR HEALTH PHASE ONE SAMPLE MENU	MANDI POINTS
BREAKFAST		**BREAKFAST**	
Blueberry muffin	0.4	Cinnamon Fruit Oatmeal	7.0
Coffee with cream and sugar	0	Orange juice	3.5
LUNCH		**LUNCH**	
McDonald's Cheeseburger	1.1	Whole-wheat pita with	
McDonald's French Fries	0.7	vegetables, avocado and	
Coke	0	Russian Fig Dressing/Dip	9.5
		Sunflower seeds	3.1
		Strawberries	7.0
SNACK			
Two chocolate chip cookies	0.3		
DINNER		**DINNER**	
Salad with iceberg lettuce and tomato	4.0	Raw vegetables	16.4
		Hummus	3.0
Lasagna with meat sauce	4.0	Pasta with Roasted	
Vanilla ice cream	0.5	Vegetables	8.5
Iced tea	0	Very Berry Ice Cream	6.0
TOTAL MANDI	**11**	**TOTAL MANDI**	**64**

SAD MENU vs. *EAT FOR HEALTH* PHASE ONE MENU

NUTRIENT	SAD SAMPLE MENU	PHASE ONE SAMPLE MENU
Calories	2057	1911
Protein %	12	12
Carbohydrate %	49	59
Fat %	39	29
Cholesterol mg	213	0
Saturated Fat g	34	9
Dietary Fiber g	17	60
Sodium mg	3811	667
Vitamin A (IU)	4523	37,585
Beta Carotene mcg	1700	18,576
Vitamin C mg	52	677
Calcium mg	785	625
Iron mg	12	19
Folate mcg	330	814
Zinc mg	7	12
TOTAL **MANDI**	**11**	**64**

AVERAGE DAILY

CALORIES	MANDI	SODIUM
1926	70	1115

[**Note:** * indicates a recipe for this listing follows]

1 DAY ONE

MANDI
75

BREAKFAST

Cinnamon Fruit Oatmeal*

Orange juice

LUNCH

Russian Fig Dressing/Dip* on Whole-wheat pita stuffed with shredded romaine, sliced tomato, chopped cucumber, and avocado slices

Strawberries

DINNER

Tossed Green Salad with dressing of choice (See purchasing guidelines on page 90 for low-fat, low-salt dressings)

Spiced Haddock or Tilapia* (Vegetarian Substitute—Chunky Sweet Potato Stew*)

Brown rice

Braised Bok Choy*

Poached Pears with Raspberry Sauce* or fresh fruit

DAY TWO

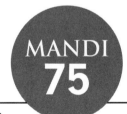

MANDI
58

BREAKFAST

Fruit and berries with plain
 or vanilla non-fat yogurt

Pomegranate juice

LUNCH

Turkey sandwich (2 oz. turkey)
 on whole-grain bread with mixed
 greens, tomato, and mustard
 (Vegetarian substitute—Eliminate
 turkey and add more vegetables,
 cashew butter or avocado)

¼ cup Sunflower Seeds

Melon and Grapes

DINNER

Raw vegetables
 (carrots, celery and red pepper)

Tasty Hummus* (Save leftover for
 Day Four lunch.)

Pasta with Roasted Vegetables*

Wild Apple Crunch* or fresh fruit

DAY THREE

MANDI
75

BREAKFAST

Grapefruit

Whole-grain toast with 100% fruit
 spread and/or nut butter

LUNCH

Orange Sesame Tossed Salad*

Fast Black Bean Soup*

Kiwi

DINNER

Hot Pepper Salsa*

Baked Garlic Pita Chips*

Turkey Spinach Burger* on whole-
 grain bun with tomato, red onion
 and lettuce (Vegetarian
 Substitute—Simple Bean Burgers*)

Sunshine Slaw*

Very Berry Ice Cream* (Easier
 Alternative—Sliced watermelon)

Note: Marinate ingredients for Mango Riesling Compote for dinner on Day Four.

DAY FOUR

MANDI 72

BREAKFAST

Whole-grain cereal with
 soy or skim milk

Blueberries

LUNCH

Tasty Hummus* (leftover from Day
 Two dinner) on whole-grain bread

Tossed green salad

Balsamic Vinaigrette* (Save
 leftover for dinner salad)

Apple

DINNER

Romaine, Spinach, and Watercress
 Salad with Fruit and Nuts*

Tomato Bean Barley Soup*
 (Save leftover for Day Five lunch)

Mango Riesling Compote
 or fresh fruit

DAY FIVE

MANDI 77

BREAKFAST

Blueberry Orange Smoothie*

LUNCH

Raw vegetables
 (carrots, cucumber, red pepper)

Bottled low-fat, low-salt dressing
 (See purchasing guidelines
 on page 90)

Tomato Bean Barley Soup* (leftover
 from Day Four dinner) or low-salt
 canned soup of your choice (See
 purchasing guidelines on page 90)

Pear

DINNER

Balsamic Mixed Greens
 with Chopped Apples*

Dijon Chicken* (Vegetarian Substitute
 – Spaghetti Squash Primavera*)

Baked Potato Fries*

California Creamed Kale*
(Easier Alternative: Lemon Zest Spinach*)

Jenna's Peach Freeze* or fresh fruit

*Note: Freeze bananas for Frozen Banana Fluff
for dinner on Day Six. Peel and freeze
bananas in a plastic bag. (This is a good way
to make sure ripe bananas don't go to waste.)*

6
DAY SIX

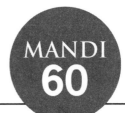

MANDI
73

BREAKFAST
Scrambled Eggs with
   Spinach and Tomatoes*

Pomegranate juice

LUNCH
Speedy Vegetable Wrap*

¼ cup raw cashew nuts

Tropical Fruit Salad*

DINNER
Raw vegetables (broccoli, carrots,
   celery, red pepper)

Garbanzo Guacamole*

Tuscan Pasta and Arugula*

Frozen Banana Fluff* (needs frozen
   bananas) or fresh fruit

*Note: If desired, freeze tofu for Marian's Tofu
Chili for dinner on Day Seven.*

7
DAY SEVEN

MANDI
60

BREAKFAST
Whole-grain bagel with
trans-fat-free "buttery" spread

Melon

LUNCH
Mixed greens, avocado and
   tomatoes with low-fat, low-salt
   dressing (See purchasing
   guidelines on page 90)

Marian's Tofu Chili*

Banana

DINNER
Artichokes with Dipping Sauce*

Steak and Roasted Vegetable Salad*
   (Vegetarian Substitute—Eliminate
   meat.)

Blueberries and strawberries

Macadamia Cream* (optional)

QUICK AND EASY MEAL SUGGESTIONS

Most of us do not cook a different dish every night for dinner; we eat some leftovers and maybe cook one thing new. If you eat like that, the weekly menu plan above may give you enough ideas, recipes and menu suggestions for two, three or even four weeks. However, you do not have to use fancy recipes all the time. Simple foods are quick and easy and can work in this program too. Consider some of the options below to make your Phase One diet easier and more convenient.

Breakfast

Combine fresh fruit in season or even frozen fruit with raw nuts and seeds, or have a hot cereal, such as oatmeal, with cut up fruit on top. Other recommended cereals are Familia Swiss Muesli (no added sugar), Wheatena, Ralston High Fiber, Roman Meal Multigrain. You could also make a quick smoothie with fruit and flax seeds, or have a hearty, whole-grain bread, like Alvarado Street, Manna Bread or Ezekiel brands, with trans-fat free spread or raw almond or cashew butter.

Lunch and Dinner

Your basic lunch should be a salad with a healthy dressing and a bowl of vegetable or bean soup that you made on the weekend. Make a quick salad from pre-mixed and pre-washed greens. Add chopped nuts, cut up fresh fruit or low-salt canned beans and use a low-fat and low-salt dressing/dip, fresh lemon, or balsamic or flavored vinegar. You can also eat raw vegetables and avocado with a low-salt salsa or hummus dip or store-bought dressing. The recommended low-calorie commercial dressings and soups can be found in the Purchasing Guidelines, on page 90.

Having some defrosted frozen vegetables, or fresh or frozen fruit is a good way to round out a meal, salad or leftover dish. Try steaming some fresh broccoli, spinach or another green vegetable and adding a flavoring like VegiZest. You can also rub down raw vegetables, such as broccoli, with a little olive oil applied to your hands and then add chopped garlic and onion. Baked potato, baked sweet potato, and corn on the cob with a trans-fat free spread or vegetable seasoning are great, easy options that are often also loved by children. A quick and tasty dish can be made from whatever fresh vegetables you have on hand.

Another easy meal option is to stuff whole-wheat pita bread or a whole wheat wrap with shredded romaine or other greens, tomato, sun dried tomatoes (pre-soaked in water), cucumber, bean sprouts, broccoli slaw, or cole slaw mix. You can add hummus, avocado, salsa, tahini, or nut butter. I often mash almond butter and tomato sauce together with Black Fig Vinegar and put it in the pita with tomatoes, avocado, and shredded lettuce. Many families enjoy whole grain lentil pasta with lots of vegetables and a good low-salt tomato sauce. Remember the knowledge that you have gained in Phase One and your meal options are endless.

EATING FOR PHASE TWO

The new recipes and menus in Phase Two are designed to have taste appeal as well as increased nutrient levels. The more you eat healthful meals and the more days you link together eating healthful foods, the more your brain will naturally prefer to eat that way. For new healthy habits to develop, you need to keep up high-nutrient eating for months. You may then be surprised to find that you actually prefer eating this way.

In this phase you will aim for a MANDI Score of 75 or better. Use the following menus or devise your own. You can incorporate some of the Phase One recipes if they are nutrient-rich. As you look through the recipes, you will begin to notice what characteristics high-scorers have in common: lots of vegetables, fruit, and beans. Recipes that include the green leafy vegetables like kale, spinach, collards and bok choy have the highest scores because these ingredients are so nutrient-dense. You can start to apply this knowledge to screening your own recipes for nutritional value.

Phase Two's recipes reflect a continued increase in high-nutrient foods and a decrease in low-nutrient foods. You may notice we have removed red meat and increased beans and nuts. We are also decreasing your salt intake to less than 1200 mg of sodium per day. Eventually this eating style will become natural to you, so hang in there.

> **HELPFUL HINT:**
> Eating too quickly encourages overeating and can tax the digestive system. It takes about 15 minutes for your brain to realize that your stomach is full. If you eat too fast, your body won't have enough time to tell you when it's full. You will end up eating more than you really needed. Slow down, thoroughly chew your food, and enjoy the experience of eating. Don't just grab food without thinking about it.

Cooking For Health

In this phase, you will prepare more high-nutrient soups. Soups and stews are critical components of this eating-style. When vegetables are simmered in soup, all the nutrients are retained in the liquid. Soups and stews are cooked at 212° F, the boiling point of water. Cooking at this low temperature is very healthful because no acrylamides are produced. Acrylamides are cancer-causing agents formed when foods are fried, baked, roasted or grilled.

Many of the soup recipes use fresh vegetable juices, especially carrot juice. These juices provide a great tasting, antioxidant-rich base. If you don't have a juicer you should consider purchasing one. If you are short of time, bottled carrot and other vegetable juices can be purchased at most health food stores, but don't expect them to taste as good as fresh squeezed. Low sodium V8 is another option to add to the soup base. The Quick and Creamy Vegetable Bean Soup recipe in this phase teaches you a simple procedure that can be used to create "cream" soups. Raw cashews or cashew butter are blended into the soup to provide a creamy texture and rich flavor. A big advantage to making soups and stews is that they are great leftovers! Soups generally keep well for up to four days in the refrigerator, but should be frozen if longer storage is desirable.

Be creative with your soup making. Once you get the general idea, you can mix and match ingredients. Start with a base like carrot juice, tomato juice or organic low-salt canned soup. (Check the Purchasing Guidelines on page 90 for brands that are low in sodium.) Add some leafy greens, a member of the onion family, some flavoring like Vegi-Zest and any other vegetables that you have on hand. Don't forget the beans! Create all new soups by matching up different items from the columns in the chart below.

SOUPS AND STEWS – THE *EAT FOR HEALTH* WAY					
BASE	**LEAFY GREENS**	**ONION FAMILY**	**OTHER VEGETABLES**	**FLAVOR**	**BEANS**
carrot juice	kale	onion	tomato, fresh/canned	VegiZest	azduki
low salt canned soup	spinach	leek	zucchini	sun dried tomato	red kidney
tomato juice	cabbage	garlic	red/green pepper	bay leaf	split peas
celery juice	Swiss chard	ginger	celery	cilantro/ parsley	black beans
Low Sodium V-8	bok choy	shallots	parsnips	chili powder/ cumin	garbanzo
beet juice	turnip greens		carrots	curry powder	lentils
	mustard greens		mushrooms	lemon	navy beans
				hot pepper	

HELPFUL HINT:

When you choose to occasionally use a prepared soup keep in mind that you want your overall daily sodium intake to remain under 1200 mg. You get around 400 to 600 mg of sodium from natural whole foods, which only leaves you with a leeway of about 600 mg. You will be amazed how much sodium canned soup contains. Be sure to read the labels.

Fish appears in the Phase Two recipes as well. Fish is a healthy source of Omega-3 fatty acids, but can also contain high levels of mercury and other toxins. Re-visit Chapter Thirteen of Book One for a list of the least and most polluted fish. The Salsa Salmon recipe on Day Two of this phase has gotten rave reviews. It's good enough for company. Choose wild over farm-raised salmon, which contains higher levels of cancer causing PCB's. The cooking style this dish features uses a small amount of animal products with lots of complimentary nutrient-rich vegetables... As you progress through the phases, animal products move from being the traditional main dish to merely an accent or flavor enhancer.

ingredient spotlight

BLUEBERRIES

Ongoing research is consistently showing that blueberries contain powerful disease-fighting compounds that may improve short-term memory, intelligence, night vision, and coordination. They also have the ability to prevent diseases such as cancer, strengthen blood capillaries, ease arthritis pain, and even slow the aging process. Blueberries have high antioxidant activity. Packed with antioxidant phytochemicals called anthocyanins, blueberries neutralize free radical damage to cells and tissues, which is linked to cancer, heart disease, Alzheimer's disease, and a range of other age-related conditions.

Blueberries were not cultivated until the beginning of the 20th century, becoming commercially available in 1916. Blueberries are native to North America, where they grow in the woods and mountainous regions of the United States and Canada. They are rarely found growing in Europe and have only recently been introduced in Australia. This miraculous little fruit can be used in a variety of breakfast dishes, smoothies, salads, and desserts.

Be Prepared

Being prepared is more than half the battle. It is those times when you get hungry and have nothing healthy to eat that you are most prone to have a setback. Always have healthful foods available for those hungry times. As you begin Phase Two, look over the menus and recipes and make a plan. Do your shopping for the week and stock up your kitchen. Don't get overwhelmed. You can choose to cook only on a few days and plan to use leftovers on the days you will be too busy. A good batch of leftovers is like money in the bank. Make a soup for dinner and use it for a second dinner or two days of lunches. A healthy dressing/dip can work on your dinner salad as well as several lunches. In a pinch refer back to the Quick and Easy Meal Suggestions at the end of Phase One.

Test your Eat For Health IQ!
Before you get started on your Phase Two menus and recipes, take this Health Equation Quiz and test how much you've learned.
(The answers are on the next page.)

1. Unprocessed foods are the key to optimal health.
   ◯ **TRUE**   ◯ **FALSE**

2. Vitamin supplements can give us all the nutrients we need.
   ◯ **TRUE**   ◯ **FALSE**

3. On the Standard American Diet (SAD), less than 10 percent of calories come from nutrient-rich foods such as fresh fruit, vegetables, beans, raw nuts and seeds.
   ◯ **TRUE**   ◯ **FALSE**

4. Dairy is the food category that contributes the most saturated fat to the Standard American Diet.
   ◯ **TRUE**   ◯ **FALSE**

5. Trans fats are the most dangerous fats to consume.
   ◯ **TRUE**   ◯ **FALSE**

6. To achieve protection from heart disease, a good goal is to have your total cholesterol below 150 and your LDL (bad) cholesterol below 100.
   ◯ **TRUE**   ◯ **FALSE**

7. Adding salt to your diet can make eating less pleasurable.
   ○ TRUE   ○ FALSE

8. If you are an athlete, you must consume more animal products to get enough high-quality protein.
   ○ TRUE   ○ FALSE

9. Eating smaller portions is the key to successful weight loss.
   ○ TRUE   ○ FALSE

10. It is better to do something imperfectly than to do nothing flawlessly.
    ○ TRUE   ○ FALSE

ANSWER KEY:

1. TRUE	2. FALSE	3. TRUE	4. TRUE	5. TRUE
6. TRUE	7. TRUE	8. FALSE	9. FALSE	10. TRUE

Nutritional Comparison

SAD MENU vs. *EAT FOR HEALTH* PHASE TWO MENU

SAD SAMPLE MENU	MANDI POINTS	EAT FOR HEALTH PHASE TWO SAMPLE MENU	MANDI POINTS
BREAKFAST		**BREAKFAST**	
Blueberry muffin	0.4	Creamy Fruit and Berry	
Coffee with cream and sugar	0	Smoothie	12.5
LUNCH		**LUNCH**	
McDonald's Cheeseburger	1.1	Raw vegetables	10.0
McDonald's French Fries	0.7	Tofu Ranch	
Coke	0	Dressing/Dip	1.5
		Portobello Red Pepper	
		Sandwich	8.0
SNACK		Grapes	1.3
Two chocolate chip cookies	0.3		
DINNER		**DINNER**	
Salad with iceberg lettuce	4.0	Romaine, Spinach,	
and tomato		and Watercress Salad	
Lasagna with meat sauce	4.0	with Fruit and Nuts	20.0
Vanilla ice cream	0.5	Quick and Creamy Vegetable	
Iced tea	0	Bean Soup	22.0
		Yummy Banana-Oat Bars	2.5
TOTAL MANDI	**11**	**TOTAL MANDI**	**78**

SAD MENU vs. *EAT FOR HEALTH* PHASE TWO MENU

Nutrient	SAD Sample Menu	Phase Two Sample Menu
Calories	2057	2017
Protein %	12	13
Carbohydrate %	49	58
Fat %	39	29
Cholesterol mg	213	0
Saturated Fat g	34	11
Dietary Fiber g	17	61
Sodium mg	3811	1022
Vitamin A (IU)	4523	54,069
Beta Carotene mcg	1700	27,072
Vitamin C mg	52	395
Calcium mg	785	942
Iron mg	12	28
Folate mcg	330	712
Zinc mg	7	11
Total **MANDI**	**11**	**78**

AVERAGE DAILY

CALORIES	MANDI	SODIUM
1855	82	973

[*Note:* * *indicates a recipe for this listing follows*]

DAY ONE

MANDI 75

BREAKFAST

Creamy Fruit and Berry Smoothie*

Orange

¼ cup sunflower seeds

LUNCH

Tasty Hummus*

Whole-wheat pita, with cucumber, romaine and tomato

Carrot sticks

Pineapple

DINNER

Mixed baby greens

Dijon Date Dressing/Dip*

Quick and Creamy Vegetable Bean Soup* (Save leftover for Day Two lunch.)

Melon

DAY TWO

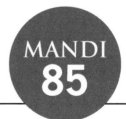

MANDI
81

BREAKFAST

Whole-grain bagel with
  trans-fat free spread

Orange juice

LUNCH

Raw vegetables
  (carrots, celery, cucumber)

Orange Cashew Dressing/Dip*

Quick and Creamy Vegetable Bean
  Soup* (Leftover from Day One
  dinner.)

Fruit and Berry Compote*

DINNER

Greens and vegetable
  with Sesame Fig Dressing*

Salsa Salmon over Wilted Greens*
  (Vegetarian Substitute—
  Southwest Vegetable Chili*)

Grapes

DAY THREE

MANDI
85

BREAKFAST

Blueberry Nut Oatmeal*

Pomegranate juice

LUNCH

Raw vegetables with leftover dip
  or low fat, low salt dressing (see
  purchasing guidelines on page 90)

2 oz. turkey on sprouted wheat
  bread with mixed greens, broccoli
  sprouts and tomato

(Vegetarian Substitute—Eliminate turkey
and add additional vegetables, almond
butter, cashew butter, or avocado.)

Strawberries

DINNER

Walnut-Pear Green Salad*

Cuban Black Beans with Brown Rice*

Fruit and Nut Bowl*

DAY FOUR

MANDI
86

BREAKFAST

Whole-grain cereal with
  soy or skim milk

Blueberries

LUNCH

Black Bean Hummus Dip*

Raw Vegetables

Gazpacho Summer Soup*
  (EASIER alternative—Avocado
  topped with salsa)

Cherries

*Note: If desired, make Banana Pumpkin
Pudding for dinner on Day Four.*

DINNER

Seasoned edamame (To cook
  edamame, put the pods in boiling
  water for 5 minutes. Drain and
  toss with Mrs. Dash or other no-
  salt seasoning. Squeeze beans
  out of shell to eat.)

Turkey-Vegetable Meatloaf*
  (Vegetarian substitute—Add beans
  to Vegetables Milanese*.)

Baked sweet potatoes

Vegetables Milanese
  (EASIER alternative—Steamed
  Broccoli and Garlic*)

Strawberries and pineapple

Chocolate Dip* (optional)

DAY FIVE

MANDI
82

BREAKFAST

Blueberry Orange Smoothie*

LUNCH

Tossed Green Salad

Balsamic Vinaigrette*

Portobello Red Pepper Sandwich

Plums

DINNER

Green Velvet Vegetable Salad*

Hearty Ginger Lentil Soup* (Save
  leftover for Day Six lunch.)

Banana Pumpkin Pudding

*Notes: Soak oats for Pomegranate Muesli for
breakfast on Day Six. Freeze bananas for
Banana Walnut Ice Cream for dinner on Day Six.*

6 DAY SIX

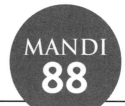

MANDI
78

BREAKFAST

Pomegranate Muesli*
  (oats need to be soaked overnight)

Orange Juice

LUNCH

Romaine wedges

Caesar Salad Dressing/Dip*

Hearty Ginger Lentil Soup*
  (Leftover from Day Five dinner)

Apple

DINNER

Red Pepper Salsa*
  with endive leaves

Creole Chicken with Spinach and
  Rice* (Vegetarian substitute—
  Replace Creole Chicken with
  Roasted Mixed Vegetables* and
  brown rice)

Banana Walnut Ice Cream* (using
  frozen bananas) or fresh fruit

7 DAY SEVEN

MANDI
88

BREAKFAST

Vegetable Omelet*

Salsa

Honeydew melon

LUNCH

Romaine, Spinach, and Watercress
  Salad with Fruit and Nuts*

Vegetable Burrito*

Kiwi

DINNER

Raw vegetables
  (cucumber, carrots, broccoli)

Tofu Ranch Dressing/Dip*

West African Lentil Okra Stew*

Yummy Banana-Oat Bars*
  or fresh fruit

EATING FOR PHASE THREE

Phase Three is a major milestone on your health makeover journey! By repeating your new behaviors over and over, they are becoming a part of you. As you eat more healthfully, you are losing your addictions to unhealthful substances and unhealthful foods.

You will now be reaching for a MANDI nutrient score of 90 or more each day. As you can probably guess, that will require further increases in your high-nutrient vegetable consumption. One of the major keys to success is to eat plenty of food, so when you eat raw or cooked greens, eat a much larger portion than you have in the past. We were not designed for deprivation when it comes to eating what nature intended for us. We need to eat large portions to ingest enough nutrients to protect our bodies from disease. Go for variety in your nutrient-dense raw and cooked vegetables and eat lots of them.

Raw vegetables can be eaten in unlimited quantities. A sensible goal is to shoot for one-pound daily. Take a small food scale and weigh a variety of vegetables: lettuce, cucumber, tomato, bell peppers, carrots, broccoli, zucchini, cauliflower, etc. You will see that one pound isn't that much. It is helpful to make up several one-pound bags of washed and prepped vegetables to carry with you or to have on hand during the week. You can add these to salads or dip them in hummus or a healthy dip as part of your meal.

With this week's meals try to get a feel for how much food you require to feel satisfied, not overly full. Keep working on getting in touch with your body's signals. Don't eat unless you are hungry. Stop eating before you are full. These concepts are very basic, but the over-processed, over-refined foods our society relies on have caused us to forget that our body has an innate intelligence to direct us to the correct amount of foods when our diet is wholesome.

At this point in your Eat For Health journey, your kitchen is set up for nutritional excellence and you have applied several cooking techniques including making nutrient-dense soups and stews and reducing oil and salt consumption by using healthy substitutions. In this phase, animal products are reduced to three servings per week, sodium levels are reduced to below 1000 mg/day, and the use of cooking oil is minimal. Oil in salad dressings and dips is replaced by making creamy dressings/dips with nutrient-rich nuts and avocados. Also, you will be introduced to nutrient-dense desserts using dates and dried fruit to satisfy your natural sweet tooth.

ingredient spotlight
DATES

Archeological findings reveal that dates have been held in high esteem since ancient times. They are one of the earliest fruits cultivated by man. The original cultivation of the date is believed to be in the Persian Gulf area or in Mesopotamia. Dates are now classed as one of the standard crops of world agriculture and are widely grown in Saudi Arabia, Egypt, Iran, Iraq, Spain, Italy, China, and the United States. Dates are rich in phosphorus, iron, and calcium, and can be eaten fresh or dried. Dehydrated and ground dates can be purchased as date sugar, which can be used as a healthier substitute for refined sugar and corn syrup.

Shopping for Phase Three

Shopping for this phase will require you to spend more time in the health food store or health food section of your supermarket. If you are not already, you will become acquainted with the bulk section. Purchasing nuts and spices from the bulk section is often less expensive than the pre-packaged variety. Remember to purchase only raw nuts and nut butters. Roasting produces harmful compounds called acrylamides and also causes a loss in nutrient value. You can use all spices and herbs except for salt. When using condiments, mustard is okay if unsalted mustard is an available option, but pickled foods contain too much salt and should be avoided. If you love ketchup or tomato sauce, you may find a lower-calorie, low-salt ketchup and tomato sauce at the health food store.

At this phase you will learn a new cooking technique that requires a lot of fresh carrots. It is a good idea to always have an ample supply of fresh carrots on hand. They will keep in the refrigerator for up to 14 days.

Salad Dressings: The *Eat For Health* Way

During this phase you will create creamy nut sauces and dressings with nuts, seeds, and avocados. *Eat For Health* is not a fat-free eating style because our bodies require healthy fats from whole foods, the way nature designed us to consume them. By eating this way, we receive the lignins, flavonoids, antioxidants, minerals, and other protective phytochemicals that come along in the package. Seeds and nuts become disease-prevention food. Salad dressings and dips usually start with oil and vinegar: the oil provides the fat and the vinegar provides the acidity. My salad dressings utilize whole foods as the fat sources: almond and cashews, other nuts and seeds, avocado, and tahini. Some popular favorites are my Caesar Salad Dressing/Dip on Day Three, the Tahini Dressing/Dip on Day Two, and a simple recipe of cashew butter with lemon juice, garlic and Dijon mustard. Gourmet fruit flavored vinegars are used in many recipes, including the Asparagus with Black Fig Vinegar, because they add unique and delicious flavors. Garlic, onions, fruit, Dijon mustard, and herbs and spices contribute additional character and interest. Items from this chart can be combined to create new flavors while maintaining the health quality of the dressings.

SALAD DRESSINGS – THE *EAT FOR HEALTH* WAY			
FLAVOR	**FAT**	**ACIDITY**	**OTHER**
Garlic	Almond Butter	Balsamic Vinegar	Tofu
Onion	Cashew Butter	Spicy Pecan Vinegar	Soy Milk
Fresh/Dried/ Frozen Fruit	Nuts/Seeds	Blood Orange Vinegar	Juice
Dijon Mustard	Avocado	Fig Vinegar	Tomato Sauce
Fresh/Dried Herbs	Tahini/Sesame Seed	Riesling Raisin Vinegar	Fruit Preserves
Spices (no salt)		D'Anjou Pear Vinegar	
VegiZest		Lemon	

Cooking for Phase Three

Vegetable juices, particularly carrot, make a robust, nutrient-dense broth for simmering vegetables. Preparing soups, stir-fries, and sautéed vegetables using this procedure is so delicious that you won't miss the salt or oil. My famous Anti-Cancer Soup is included in Phase Three and uses both juicing and blending techniques to help us approach the pinnacle of nutritional health. Don't listen to those who say that it is not possible to cook delicious food without salt or oil. My unique culinary techniques allow you to eliminate unhealthy fats and sodium while also increasing the nutrient-density of every dish, and just as important, this food tastes great.

Eating is meant to be pleasurable and an attractive food presentation enhances your dining experience. Pay attention to the colors of the fruits and vegetables. Use the seasons to inspire a color scheme. For example, a carrot juice base soup becomes a beautiful autumn red color by adding a cut-up beet to the soup. Using chopped fresh parsley or herbs, chopped nuts, and seeds to sprinkle over dishes will add beauty and flavor while also increasing the nutrients. You can experience the vibrant colors of health first hand.

> **HELPFUL HINT:**
> The quality of the food is what makes the dish. You can have the most incredible combination of seasonings and superb preparation, but if the quality of the ingredients is poor, the dish will miss the mark. The most simple of foods are delicious as long as the ingredients are top quality. Don't skimp on quality or freshness.

Quickie Quiz

1. In the history of nutritional science, one of the only things conclusively proven to dramatically and consistently extend lifespan is:

    ⃝A Adequate dietary protein

    ⃝B A vitamin and mineral supplement

    ⃝C Caloric restriction with nutrient adequacy

    ⃝D The Mediterranean diet

2. To get in touch with the amount of calories your body really needs you should:

   ○**A** Reduce portions and count calories

   ○**B** Eat before you feel hungry

   ○**C** Eat when you feel true hunger

   ○**D** Eat frequent small meals

3. Phytochemicals are:

   ○**A** Plant fertilizer

   ○**B** Essential micronutrients, not typically found in vitamin pills

   ○**C** Fragile chemicals naturally present in plants

   ○**D** B and C

4. Saturated fats are:

   ○**A** Solid at room temperature

   ○**B** A contributory cause of heart disease and cancer

   ○**C** Found mostly in meat and dairy

   ○**D** All of the above

5. The following statement about sodium is false:

   ○**A** Any excess salt added to food, outside of what is contained in natural foods, will likely increase your risk of developing high blood pressure.

   ○**B** High blood pressure and the resultant strokes are not observed in populations that do not use salt.

   ○**C** Using too much sodium causes you to lose appreciation for the natural and subtle flavors of food.

   ○**D** Although iodized salt is known to raise blood pressure and increase risk of stroke, natural salts like sea salt and organic Celtic salt do not have this effect.

ANSWER KEY:

1. C   2. C   3. D.   4. D   5. D

Nutritional Comparison

SAD MENU vs. *EAT FOR HEALTH* PHASE THREE MENU

SAD SAMPLE MENU	MANDI POINTS	EAT FOR HEALTH PHASE THREE SAMPLE MENU	MANDI POINTS
BREAKFAST		**BREAKFAST**	
Blueberry muffin	0.4	Egg and	
Coffee with cream and sugar	0	Vegetable Scramble	21.0
		Avocado	2.6
		Honeydew	1.8
LUNCH		**LUNCH**	
McDonald's Cheeseburger	1.1	Raw vegetables	8.0
McDonald's French Fries	0.7	Caesar Salad	
Coke	0	Dressing/Dip	1.5
		Roasted Vegetable Pizza	20.0
		Apple	2.5
SNACK		Raw nuts or nut butter	1.6
Two chocolate chip cookies	0.3		
DINNER		**DINNER**	
Salad with iceberg lettuce and tomato	4.0	Tossed Salad with Dijon Pistachio Dressing	13.0
Lasagna with meat sauce	4.0	Eggplant Roulades	16.5
Vanilla ice cream	0.5	Banana Fig Ice Cream	2.0
Iced tea	0		
TOTAL MANDI	**11**	**TOTAL MANDI**	**91**

SAD MENU vs. *EAT FOR HEALTH* PHASE THREE MENU

NUTRIENT	SAD SAMPLE MENU	PHASE THREE SAMPLE MENU
Calories	2057	1964
Protein %	12	16
Carbohydrate %	49	50
Fat %	39	34
Cholesterol mg	213	423
Saturated Fat g	34	13
Dietary Fiber g	17	70
Sodium mg	3811	991
Vitamin A (IU)	4523	76,410
Beta Carotene mcg	1700	41,194
Vitamin C mg	52	673
Calcium mg	785	998
Iron mg	12	28
Folate mcg	330	1477
Zinc mg	7	12
TOTAL **MANDI**	**11**	**91**

AVERAGE DAILY		
CALORIES	**MANDI**	**SODIUM**
1922	93	856

*[**Note:** * indicates a recipe for this listing follows]*

1 DAY ONE

MANDI
88

BREAKFAST
Banana-Cashew Lettuce Wrap*

Low-sodium vegetable juice

LUNCH
Vegetable Garbanzo Wrap*

Broccoli Vinaigrette*

Mango

DINNER
Tossed Salad with Dijon
  Pistachio Dressing*

Speedy Vegetable and Bean Soup*
  (Save leftover for Day Two lunch.)

Strawberries, blueberries
  and banana

Strawberry Dressing*

*Note: Soak Fruit Compote overnight for
breakfast on Day Two.*

DAY TWO

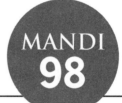

MANDI
94

BREAKFAST

Oatmeal and Fruit Compote*

LUNCH

Raw vegetables
(broccoli, red pepper)

Tahini Dressing/Dip*
(save leftover for dinner salad)

Speedy Vegetable and Bean Soup*
(Leftover from Day One dinner.)

Grapes

DINNER

Mixed Greens

Tahini Dressing/Dip*

Thai Vegetable Curry*.

Fresh fruit

*Note: Freeze bananas for Mixed Berry
Freeze for dinner on Day Three.*

DAY THREE

MANDI
98

BREAKFAST

Chocolate Smoothie*

LUNCH

Mixed greens, avocado, and
tomatoes with low-fat, low-salt
dressing (See purchasing guidelines
on page 90)

Roasted Vegetable Pizza*

Apple

DINNER

Raw vegetables
(carrots, red pepper, broccoli)

Caesar Salad Dressing/Dip*

Southwestern Chicken*
(Vegetarian substitute—Quick
Vegetable Bean Medley*)

Cauliflower Spinach Mashed
"Potatoes"* (EASIER alternative—
Steamed Asparagus)

Mixed Berry Freeze*
(need frozen bananas) or fresh fruit

DAY FOUR

MANDI 89

BREAKFAST

Special Oatmeal*

Pomegranate juice

LUNCH

Whole-wheat pita stuffed with
shredded romaine, sliced tomato,
broccoli sprouts, and avocado
slices

Tomato Almond Dressing/Dip*

Healthy Slaw*

Cherries

DINNER

Citrus Salad
with Orange Peanut Dressing*

Dr. Fuhrman's Famous
Anti-Cancer Soup*
(Save leftovers for Day Five lunch)

Melon

DAY FIVE

MANDI 90

BREAKFAST

Sprouted grain bread with
raw nut butter

Banana

LUNCH

Asparagus with Black Fig Dressing*

Dr. Fuhrman's Famous Anti-Cancer
Soup* (Leftover from Day Four
dinner)

Blueberries

DINNER

Tossed green salad

Balsamic Vinaigrette*

¼ cup chopped walnuts

Eggplant Roulades*

Bluevado Pie* or fresh fruit

Note: Freeze bananas for Banana Fig Ice
Cream for dinner on Day Six.

DAY SIX

MANDI
96

BREAKFAST

Lisa's Favorite Green Smoothie*

¼ cup pecans

LUNCH

Southern-Style Mixed Greens*

Brussels Sprouts Polonaise*

Pear

DINNER

Tossed green salad with avocado slices and low-fat, low-salt dressing of choice (See purchasing guidelines on page 90)

Black Forest Cream of Mushroom Soup* (Save leftover for Day Seven lunch.)

Banana Fig Ice Cream* (need frozen bananas) or fresh fruit

DAY SEVEN

MANDI
99

BREAKFAST

Egg and Vegetable Scramble*

Sprouted grain bread, toasted

LUNCH

Greens and Berries Salad with Cashew Currant Dressing*

Black Forest Cream of Mushroom Soup* (Leftover from Day Six dinner)

DINNER

Crazy-About-Carrot Salad*

Pasta with Shrimp and Artichokes* (Vegetarian substitute—Vegetable Shepherd's Pie*)

Nutrient-Rich Chocolate Pudding* or fresh fruit

Note: Nutrient-Rich Chocolate Pudding needs to be made ahead of time and chilled.

Focusing on the Final Phase

Congratulations! After completing the first three phases of this book, your health makeover is well underway. You now have the knowledge to make better decisions about the kind of diet you eat. Take some time to assess how you are feeling. Toxic withdrawal symptoms should be behind you. Your food preferences should be changing as you experience how tasty high-nutrient eating can be. By stripping away excess salt, artificial flavors, refined sugars and sweeteners, and empty-calorie fats you are giving your body the opportunity to enjoy a whole spectrum of natural flavors that you may have never appreciated.

Have you been getting in touch with true hunger? Have you stopped eating before you are full? Remember, the next meal is more enjoyable when you don't overeat at the prior meal and you can eat whenever you feel hungry again. As a species we have evolved to store up calories in case of famine. There is no longer any immediate danger of that happening. It's ok to let yourself get hungry. It makes food taste better when you eat!

In this phase, we will move on to how to disease-proof yourself and how to recover from a medical condition by mastering the most nutrient-dense food preparations: raw food blending, juicing, and cruciferous soup making. In this final phase, the goal is to get your nutrient score over 100. The daily sodium level has been reduced to below 900 mg/day and there are only two servings per week of animal products.

Cooking For Phase Four

To maximize the nutrient density of your diet, daily consumption of a thick vegetable soup or stew is recommended. Soups and stews can be made in advance in large amounts so they are readily available the entire week. By blending a portion of it, you not only create a delicious creamy and chunky soup, you also make the nutrients more absorbable. Phase Four recipes feature several nutrient-dense soups and stews for you to practice with. The High Cruciferous Vegetable Stew we feature in the Day One menu achieved a MANDI score of 34,which makes a significant contribution toward your daily goal of 100 points.

Blending raw vegetables with fruit is an efficient way to increase your nutrient absorption. When we normally eat a salad, the majority of the micronutrients do not get absorbed because the cell walls are not adequately crushed. In contrast, when you make creamy-tasting, high-nutrient fruit and vegetable smoothies, the absorption of beneficial phytochemicals is increased over 500 percent. They supply you with a dynamite nutrient punch and are incredibly satisfying. As mentioned, you may want to consider investing in a high-performance blender.

Blending a mixture of raw, leafy greens and other ingredients makes a smooth, creamy cold soup or smoothie. By adding fruit you can satisfy your natural sweet tooth. The term blended salad or green smoothie refers to the technique of combining raw vegetables, fruit and other ingredients to make a highly absorbable salad which can be consumed at breakfast or with any meal. The Eat Your Greens Fruit Smoothie, for example, blends fresh spinach with banana, blueberries, and pomegranate juice. There are infinite blending combinations. In Phase Four, we give you several options and encourage you to make your own combinations of anything from creamy cold vegetable soups to pudding-like desserts. Start with some greens, like spinach, kale, romaine or avocado. Add in some fresh or frozen fruit, such as blueberries, strawberries, oranges, banana, pineapple, kiwi. You can also add other flavors and liquids according to your taste preferences. This chart will help you come up with new possibilities.

SMOOTHIES – THE *EAT FOR HEALTH* WAY			
LIQUID (*optional*)	GREENS	FRUIT (*Fresh or Frozen*)	FLAVOR/OTHER
Almond or Soy Milk	Spinach	Blueberries	Dates
Pomegranate Juice	Avocado	Strawberries	Flax Seed
Orange Juice	Kale	Oranges	Goji Berries
Pineapple Juice	Lettuce	Banana	Cocoa Powder, natural
Other Fruit Juices	Cucumber	Pineapple	Nuts

In addition to blending, this phase also introduces several recipes for nutrient-dense juices including the Mixed Vegetable Juice and the Raw Vegetable Cruciferous Juice. With juicing, you retain many of the phytochemicals and other nutrients but lose other beneficial components like fiber and proteins. Juicing should not replace the fruits or vegetables in your diet, but it is an effective way to boost your nutrient absorption because you can consume a lot of nutrients from raw green vegetables easily. Some people have difficulty digesting large quantities of roughage when they first switch to a natural, plant-based diet. Often problems with gas and bloating can be solved by replacing some whole, raw, and cooked fruits and vegetables with blended dishes and juices.

HELPFUL HINT:
The cruciferous vegetables include kale, bok choy, cabbage, cauliflower, broccoli, broccoli rabe, broccoli sprouts, brussel sprouts, mustard greens, watercress, turnip greens, cauliflower, collards, arugula and radishes. Since cruciferous vegetables are your best weapons against cancer, we have included several cruciferous vegetable soups and stew recipes. Eat a good portion of these vegetables every day and sneak them into every recipe you can!

In addition to the great smoothies and juices in Phase Four, other stand-out recipes include the No Pasta Vegetable Lasagna, the Greek Chickpea Salad, and the Asian Vegetable Stir-Fry. Try to explore foods and grocery stores from different cultures on this stage of your journey. You will often be rewarded with new nutrient-dense produce that will keep your menu fresh and different. Now that you are well into Phase Four make sure you treat yourself to our wonderful Healthy Chocolate Cake. You will be amazed how these healthy ingredients can come together to provide such a great dessert.

How to Keep Going

The cooking instructions here are intended to encourage you to branch out with your own creative recipes. Many people who follow these guidelines, as a result of reading my earlier book, Eat To Live, have been experimenting and sharing delightful high-nutrient recipes on my website. However, this lifestyle does not have to be complicated. You may spend far less time in the kitchen than before. It is so easy to just shred some romaine lettuce and drizzle some tahini and lemon juice over it, heat up a tasty vegetable stew, or make a green smoothie. The nice outcome of eating this way is that even simple foods will taste better.

Don't forget to make creative use of leftovers. You do not need to cook every day. Plan to cook a healthy, nutrient-dense soup or stew two times a week. The leftovers can be used for lunch or dinners in the days that follow. The same can be done with dips and salad dressings.

ingredient spotlight
TOFU

. . . .

Some of you may be unfamiliar with tofu. Tofu is a soybean derivative, a soft, cheese-like food made by curdling liquefied soybeans. The curds then are generally pressed into a solid block like cheese. Tofu is rich in high-quality protein and low in saturated fat and sodium. Two types of tofu are available in most supermarkets: firm and silken. Firm tofu is dense and solid and holds up well in stir-fry dishes, stews, and soups. Silken tofu is made by a slightly different process that results in a creamy, custard-like product. It works well in pureed or blended dishes and makes great creamy sauces. All tofu acts like a sponge and has the ability to soak up any flavor. Crumble it into a pot of chili sauce and it tastes like chili. Blend it with cocoa and dates and it becomes a double for chocolate cream pie filling. Freeze it for a meaty texture. Cubes of firm tofu can be added to almost any dish.

Tofu is sold in water-filled tubs, vacuum packs, or in aseptic brick package. Leftover tofu should be rinsed and covered with fresh water for storage. Change the water daily to keep it fresh, and use the tofu within a week. Tofu can also be frozen. Defrosted tofu has a pleasant caramel color and a chewier, spongier texture compared to fresh. The soft consistency of tofu and its mild taste make it a good food choice for anyone. Particularly, it is a good source of protein for elderly people who prefer dishes that are easy to chew and digest.

. . . .

The following plan is a guide for you to create your own menus that include all the required nutrients for optimal health:

SAMPLE DAILY MENU PLAN

BREAKFAST

Green Smoothie
or
Fresh fruit with nuts, seeds or avocado

LUNCH

Vegetable bean soup
Green salad with fruit on top

DINNER

Salad with chopped raw vegetables
Steamed vegetables with a sauce
Fruit or one of the Eat For Health desserts
or
Salad
Vegetable main dish
Fruit or one of the Eat For Health desserts

Don't forget that an important key to success is to make a commitment to take the time each week to plan your menu and shopping list. After you finish reading, experimenting with and eating the Phase Four menus and recipes, you are ready to try to create a menu plan on your own. Pick your favorite recipes from any of the phases here and combine them with some quick and simple dishes. Set aside two times per week to cook and prepare the food for the entire week. Your final assignment is to organize your own menu and shopping list for Phase Five—the rest of your life. Use recipes from this book that you like, visit www.DrFuhrman.com for more options or use my other books and publications as an additional source of healthy recipes. It helps to keep a file or list of your favorite recipes to make menu planning faster and easier.

The time you have spent on transforming your health will bring you benefits for years to come. As you continue your body makeover, I would be thrilled to hear about how your life and health have changed. I hope you have a pleasurable journey on your path to a long and healthy life.

NUTRITIONAL COMPARISON

SAD MENU vs. *EAT FOR HEALTH* PHASE FOUR MENU

SAD SAMPLE MENU	MANDI POINTS	EAT FOR HEALTH PHASE FOUR SAMPLE MENU	MANDI POINTS
BREAKFAST		**BREAKFAST**	
Blueberry muffin	0.4	Eat Your Greens	
Coffee with cream and sugar	0	Fruit Smoothie	18.0
		Orange	3.6
LUNCH		**LUNCH**	
McDonald's Cheeseburger	1.1	Mixed Greens and Fruit	
McDonald's French Fries	0.7	w/ Blueberry Dressing	28
Coke	0	High Cruciferous	
		Vegetable Stew	34.0
SNACK			
Two chocolate chip cookies	0.3		
DINNER		**DINNER**	
Salad with iceberg lettuce and tomato	4.0	Indian Mango Salad	5.5
		Asian Vegetable Stir-Fry	24.5
Lasagna with meat sauce	4.0	Apple Surprise	5.5
Vanilla ice cream	0.5		
Iced tea	0		
TOTAL MANDI	**11**	**TOTAL MANDI**	**119**

SAD MENU vs. *EAT FOR HEALTH* PHASE FOUR MENU

NUTRIENT	SAD SAMPLE MENU	PHASE FOUR SAMPLE MENU
Calories	2057	1661
Protein %	12	14
Carbohydrate %	49	65
Fat %	39	21
Cholesterol mg	213	0
Saturated Fat g	34	9
Dietary Fiber g	17	77
Sodium mg	3811	478
Vitamin A (IU)	4523	82,525
Beta Carotene mcg	1700	45,281
Vitamin C mg	52	899
Calcium mg	785	1337
Iron mg	12	32
Folate mcg	330	1717
Zinc mg	7	13
TOTAL **MANDI**	**11**	**119**

AVERAGE DAILY		
CALORIES 1800	MANDI 114	SODIUM 639

[*Note:* * *indicates a recipe for this listing follows*]

DAY ONE

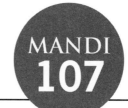

MANDI
107

BREAKFAST

Quick Banana Breakfast To Go*

LUNCH

Raw vegetables
  (broccoli, carrots, and red pepper)

Russian Fig Dressing/Dip*

Black Bean Lettuce Bundles*

Melon

DINNER

Quinoa Bean Salad*

High Cruciferous Vegetable Stew*
  (Save leftover for Day Two lunch.)

Apple Surprise* or fresh fruit

DAY TWO

MANDI
105

BREAKFAST

Eat Your Greens Fruit Smoothie*

¼ cup sunflower seeds

LUNCH

Greek Chickpea Salad*

High Cruciferous Vegetable Stew*
  (Leftover from Day One dinner)

Mixed Berries

DINNER

Indian Mango Salad*

Asian Vegetable Stir-Fry*

Sliced pineapple

DAY THREE

MANDI
107

BREAKFAST

Mixed Vegetable Juice* (Note: This
  recipe requires a juicer.)

Special Oatmeal*

LUNCH

Mixed Greens and Fruit
  with Blueberry Dressing*

French Minted Pea Soup*

DINNER

Tossed green salad
  with dressing recipe of choice

Spaghetti Squash Primavera*

Orange Sesame Kale*

Berry Cobbler* or fresh fruit

DAY FOUR

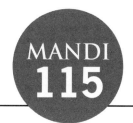

MANDI
112

BREAKFAST

Chocolate Smoothie*

Orange

LUNCH

Eggplant Hummus* on Whole-grain
tortilla with tomato, romaine, and
chopped red pepper

Raisin Coleslaw*

Super Nut Mix (1/4 cup Brazil nuts,
walnuts, and pecans)

Apple

DINNER

Asparagus Shiitake Salad
with Creamy Sesame Dressing*

Hearty Vegetable Stew*
(Save leftover for Day Five lunch.)

Strawberry Pineapple Sorbet*
with sliced strawberries or fresh
fruit

DAY FIVE

MANDI
115

BREAKFAST

High Cruciferous Juice*
(Note: This recipe requires a juicer.)

Whole-grain bread

Nut butter

Raspberries

LUNCH

Greens and Brown Rice Salad
with Pine Nuts, Apples and
Currents*

Hearty Vegetable Stew*
(Leftover from Day Four dinner)

Watermelon

DINNER

Seasoned edamame

Garden Stuffed Vegetables*

Hawaiian Sweet Potato Pudding*

DAY SIX

MANDI 118

BREAKFAST
Creamy Greeny Blended Salad*

Grapefruit

LUNCH
Mishmash Salad
   with Orange Cashew Dressing*

Spinach and
   Brussels Sprouts Delight*

Plums

DINNER
Raw vegetables (broccoli, carrots,
   celery and red pepper)

Tofu Ranch Dressing/Dip*

Filet of Sole with Mango Salsa*
   (Vegetarian Substitute—
   Scrambled Tofu*)

Chard and Vegetable Medley*

Strawberries and blueberries

DAY SEVEN

MANDI 133

BREAKFAST
Pomegranate juice

Garden Eggs and Tofu with Salsa*

Tropical Fruit Salad*

LUNCH
Broccoli with Red Lentil Sauce*
   on mixed greens

Raisin Collards and Carrots*

Cherries

DINNER
Raw vegetables (carrots, cucumber,
   red pepper)

Spicy Bean Dressing/Dip*

No Pasta Vegetable Lasagna*

Healthy Chocolate Cake*

Note: If you are pressed for time, substitute another manual dessert for the Healthy Chocolate Cake.

ANDI AND MANDI SCORES
OF COMMONLY EATEN FOODS

ANDI scores rate foods on a scale of 1 – 1000.

MANDI scores assign point values to specific serving sizes
of foods and recipes.
Use MANDI scores when rating your daily menu.

VEGETABLES

	ANDI	SERVING SIZE	MANDI
Mustard Greens, cooked	1000	1.5 cups	25.0
Watercress, raw	1000	3 cups	7.0
Kale, cooked	1000	1.5 cups	25.0
Turnip Greens, cooked	1000	1.5 cups	25.0
Collard Greens, cooked	1000	1.5 cups	33.0
Bok Choy, cooked	819	1.5 cups	20.5
Spinach, raw	738	5 cups	18.5
Spinach, cooked	702	1.5 cups	23.0
Swiss Chard, cooked	670	1.5 cups	16.7
Brussels Sprouts	667	2 cups	22.0
Arugula, raw	556	5 cups	9.5
Radish	550	7 items	2.2
Bean Sprouts	441	1 cup	11.0
Cabbage, raw	402	1.5 cups	10.1
Romaine	384	5 cups	9.6

Vegetable Juice	367	8 oz	9.1
Broccoli, raw	361	1.5 cups	9.0
Zucchini	355	2.5 cups (1 item)	8.9
Boston Lettuce	353	5 cups	8.8
Carrot Juice	346	1 cup	14.2
Dandelion Greens, cooked	334	1.5 cups	8.4
Tomato Sauce	332	½ cup	5.6
Red Pepper	332	1.5 cups	8.3
Broccoli, cooked	330	2 cups	13.5
Escarole, raw	321	3 cups	5.5
Carrots, raw	292	1.5 cups	7.6
Cauliflower	284	1.5 cups	7.1
Green Pepper	255	1.5 cups	6.4
Asparagus	233	2.0 cups	8.0
Salsa	227	¼ cup	2.5
Tomato, diced	168	2 cups	5.6
Butternut Squash	158	1.5 cups	7.8
Mushrooms	128	1.5 cups	3.2
Beets	126	1.5 cups	4.0
Celery	124	1.5 cups	1.7
Iceberg Lettuce	109	5 cups	2.7
Eggplant	98	2 cups	3.2
Sweet Potato	82	1 cup	4.4
Green Peas	75	1.5 cups	4.1
Artichoke	64	2 items	2.1
Onions	50	1 cup	1.6
Cucumber	49	1 item	1.2
Potato	34	1.5 cups	1.8
Corn	24	1.5 cups	1.5

FRUIT

	ANDI	SERVING SIZE	MANDI
Strawberries	211	1.5 cups	7.0
Pomegranate Juice	172	4 oz	5.7
Plums	156	3 items	6.4
Raspberries	146	1.5 cups	6.0
Blueberries	128	1.5 cups	6.3
Grapefruit	128	1.5 cups	5.3
Orange	108	1 item	3.6
Cantaloupe	99	2 cups	4.1
Kiwi	98	2 items	4.0
Watermelon	90	2.5 cups	3.7
Orange Juice	86	8 oz	3.5
Apple	75	1 item	2.5
Peach	74	2 items	2.4
Cherries	68	1.5 cups	3.3
Apricots	65	4 items	2.1
Pineapple	64	1.5 cups	2.6
Mango	51	1 item	2.5
Prunes	46	¼ cup	1.9
Pears	45	1 item	1.9
Honeydew Melon	44	2 cups	2.2
Avocado	37	half	2.6
Grapes	31	1.5 cups	1.3
Banana	30	1 item	1.2
Figs	29	¼ cup	1.2
Dates	19	¼ cup	0.9
Raisins	16	¼ cup	0.7

NUTS

	ANDI	SERVING SIZE	MANDI
Brazil Nuts	116	¼ cup	6.8
Sunflower Seeds	53	¼ cup	3.1
Flax Seeds	43	2 T	1.4
Sesame Seeds	40	¼ cup	2.4
Pumpkin Seeds	35	¼ cup	1.9
Pecans	33	¼ cup	1.8
Tahini Butter	29	2 T	1.6
Walnuts	29	¼ cup	1.6
Pistachios	28	¼ cup	1.5
Almonds	25	¼ cup	1.5
Peanuts	19	¼ cup	1.1
Peanut Butter	18	2 T	1.0
Cashews	15	¼ cup	0.8
Cashew Butter	13	2 T	0.7
Pine Nuts	11	¼ cup	0.6
Macadamias	10	¼ cup	0.6

BEANS

	ANDI	SERVING SIZE	MANDI
Tofu	85	4 oz	2.8
Lentils	68	1 cup	4.0
Black Beans	57	1 cup	3.4
Edamame	57	1 cup	3.7
Adzuki Beans	55	1 cup	3.5
Kidney Beans	55	1 cup	3.3

Soybeans	47	1 cup	3.0
Chickpeas	47	1 cup	3.0
Soy Burgers	42	1 item	2.1
Soy Milk	40	8 oz	2.0
Soy Cheese	27	½ cup	1.5

GRAINS

	ANDI	SERVING SIZE	MANDI
Oats, cooked	53	1 cup	3.1
Brown Rice, cooked	40	1 cup	2.4
Sprouted Grain Bread	39	1 slice	2.3
Barley, cooked	32	1 cup	1.7
Whole Wheat Bread	24	1 slice	.8
Quinoa, cooked	21	1 cup	1.1
Whole Wheat Pasta, cooked	19	2 cups	1.3
White Pasta, cooked	18	2 cups	1.3
White Bread	17	1 slice	0.9
Bagel, whole grain	18	1 item	1.0
White Rice, cooked	12	1 cup	0.7

FISH

	ANDI	SERVING SIZE	MANDI
Yellow fin Tuna	45	3 oz	2.5
Flounder/Sole	40	3 oz	2.0
Shrimp	40	3 oz	1.3
Salmon	39	3 oz	1.9
Swordfish	38	3 oz	2.0
Canned Tuna, in water	35	3 oz	1.7
Cod	32	3 oz	1.1

DAIRY

	ANDI	SERVING SIZE	MANDI
Skim Milk	36	8 oz	1.2
Plain Yogurt, low fat	26	1 cup	1.4
Feta Cheese	21	2 oz	1.1
Whole Milk	20	8 oz	1.0
Cottage Cheese, low fat	18	1 cup	1.0
Fruit Yogurt, low fat	14	1 cup	0.9
Cheddar Cheese	11	2 oz	0.6
American Cheese	10	2 oz	0.6
Vanilla Frozen Yogurt	9	1 cup	0.5
Vanilla Ice Cream	7	1 cup	0.5
Cream Cheese	4	4 tablespoons	0.2

MEAT

	ANDI	SERVING SIZE	MANDI
Deli Turkey Breast	33	3 oz (3 slices)	1.1
Eggs	28	2 items	1.4
Chicken Breast	27	3 oz	1.3
London Broil	26	3 oz	1.6
Pork Loin	23	3 oz	1.4
Ground Beef	20	3 oz	1.3
Bologna	13	3 oz (3 slices)	0.7
Hot Dog, beef	8	1 item	0.4

REFINED/PROCESSED

	ANDI	SERVING SIZE	MANDI
Milk Chocolate Bar	21	1 bar (43g)	1.3
Pizza	18	2 slices	1.2
McDonalds Cheeseburger	16	1 item	1.0
Popcorn	14	4 cups	0.7
Pretzels	13	10 items	0.8
Potato Chips	11	1 oz (10 items	0.6
Saltine Crackers	11	5 items	0.4
Granola Bars, Chocolate Chip	11	1 item	0.4
McDonalds French Fries	10	medium bag	0.7
Sugar Cookies	5	2 items	0.2
Corn Oil	3	1 Tablespoon	0.1
Olive Oil	3	1 Tablespoon	0.1
Honey	1	1 Tablespoon	0.0
Cola	0.7	8 oz	0.0

A DESCRIPTION OF THE ANDI AND MANDI NUTRIENT SCORING SYSTEM

Dr. Fuhrman's Aggregate Nutrient Density Index (ANDI):
Nutrient Data for each food item was obtained for an equal caloric amount of each food. The following nutrients were included in the evaluation:

Vitamin C

Calcium

Iron

Vitamin E

Thiamin

Riboflavin

Niacin

Vitamin B12

Vitamin B6

Folate

Magnesium

Zinc

Selenium

Dietary Fiber (total)

Carotenoids:

      Beta Carotene

      Alpha Carotene

      Lutein and Zeaxanthin

      Lycopene

Glucosinolate – compounds from cruciferous vegetables

ORAC score – Oxygen Radical Absorbance Capacity is a method of measuring the antioxidant or radical scavenging capacity of foods.

Nutrient quantities were converted to a percentage of their RDI. Since there is currently no RDI for Carotenoids, Glucosinolates, or ORAC score, the following goals were established, for the purpose of these calculations, based on available research and current understanding of the benefits of these factors:

Carotenoids[1]:

Beta Carotene 6.0 mg
Alpha Carotene 1.5 mg
Lutein and Zeaxanthin 4.2 mg
Lycopene 6.5 mg

Glucosinolates[2]:

Ten servings per week of cruciferous vegetables was considered to be optimal. It was determined that on average, 10 servings per week would translate to a daily intake of 35 mg glucosinolates. That was set as the goal for these calculations.

ORAC[3]:

Evidence suggests that daily intake should be between 3000–5000 ORAC units to have significant impact on plasma and tissue antioxidant capacity. A daily goal of 5000 ORAC units was chosen as the goal for these calculations.

The percent RDI or goal for each nutrient was added together to give a total for each food item. (The ORAC score was given a weight of 2 due to the importance of antioxidant nutrients.)

Since the total for kale was at or near the top of all commonly consumed foods that number was multiplied by .02472 to make kale's total score = 1000. This factor was determined by the formula 1000/total nutrient value of kale. Each food's total nutrient value was then multiplied by this same factor of .02472, so that they would be all scored on a 1 to 1000 scale, where kale equals 1000. Where possible, values for calories, and all nutrients other then Glucosinolate and ORAC were obtained from the USDA Database for Standard Reference.[4] In a few cases, nutrient values from foods of similar composition were used to supply missing data.

Glucosinolate and ORAC scores were obtained from the best available sources.[5,6] In some cases ORAC values were estimated using values of similar foods. It should be noted that nutrient values have variations due to soil type, season, geography, genetics, animal diets, processing, method of preparation, changes in product formulations, sampling designs, and methods of analysis.

Dr. Fuhrman's Menu Aggregate Nutrient Density Index (MANDI):
MANDI is a food, meal and menu scoring system which assigns point values to specific serving sizes of individual foods and recipes. The purpose is to guide people towards achieving an ideal MANDI of 100 points per day. It is an aid to help visualize how to choose a diet rich in micronutrients. MANDI Scores for recipes were rounded to simplify menu calculations.

---

1. Food and Nutrition Board, Institute of Medicine. Dietary Reference Intakes for Vitamin C, Vitamin E, Selenium and Carotenoids; National Academy Press, Washington D.C. 2000; 4026-4037.

2. Higdon J. Isothiocyanates; 2005; The Linus Pauling Institute, Micronutrient Research Center.

3. McBride J. Can Foods Forestall Aging? Agricultural Research 1999; 47(2): 15-17.

4. Nutritionist Pro Nutrition Analysis Software, Versions 2.5, 3.1, Axxya Systems, Stafford TX, 2005, 2006.

5. Wu X, Beecher G, Holden J, et al. Lipophilic and Hydrophilic Antioxidant Capacities of Common Foods in the United States Journal of Agricultural and Food Chemistry 2004; 52:4026-4037.

6. See Reference 2.

The equation to determine the MANDI score is:

MANDI = ANDI/1000 x Calorie factor

CALORIE RANGE	CALORIE FACTOR
1-4	1
5-9	4
10-14	7
15-19	11
20-24	14
25-29	17
30 - 59	25
60 - 89	33
90 -119	41
120 - 149	49
150 - 199	54
200 - 249	59
250 - 299	64
300 and up	69

Here are some guidelines for purchasing ready-made salad dressings, soups, tomato products and beans. Prepared commercial foods are typically high in sodium, so read the label carefully.

Some products that meet these guidelines are listed. If they can't be found in your local supermarket or health food store, most of these companies have online stores where you can order their products.

SALAD DRESSINGS

General Guidelines per two Tablespoon serving: Less than 200 mg of Sodium

	CALORIES	SODIUM
Annie's Naturals		
Low-Fat Mustard Vinaigrette	45	200
Low-Fat Raspberry Vinaigrette	35	75
A Perfect Pear		
Ginger Pear Salad Dressing	20	0
Consorzio		
Mango Dressing	30	10
Raspberry and Balsamic Dressing	30	0
Strawberry Balsamic	20	0
Kozlowski Farms		
Honey Mustard	30	105
Spicy Mexican	10	180
Zesty Herb	10	160
Raspberry Poppy	15	85
Sesame Seed	15	190

Maple Grove Farms

Fat-Free Raspberry Vinaigrette	35	180
Fat-Free Honey Dijon	40	200
Fat-Free Balsamic Vinaigrette	5	160
Fat-Free Cranberry Vinaigrette	20	180
Fat-Free Poppy Seed	40	80
Fat-Free Lime Basil Vinaigrette	25	90
Fat-Free Wasabi Dijon	35	200
Fat-Free Vidalia	20	140

Tres Classic

Grand Garlic	5	95
Caesar	10	60
Lemon Dijon	5	100
Cabernet Herb	16	0
Honey Dijon	20	110
Red Raspberry	20	0
Tomato Herb French	15	5

Walden Farms

Thousand Island	0	190
Red Wine Vinaigrette	0	190
Classic French	0	180
Russian	0	190

SOUPS

General Guidelines per one cup of soup: Less than 200 mg of Sodium

	CALORIES	SODIUM
Pacific Natural Foods		
Low Sodium Organic Veg Broth	15	140
Imagine		
Low Sodium Organic Veg Broth	20	140
Health Valley Soup - No salt added, organic		
Black Bean	130	25
Lentil	100	25
Minestrone	70	45
Tomato	80	35
Vegetable	80	40
Mushroom Barley	70	25
Potato Leek	70	45
Split Pea	110	115

BEANS

General Guidelines for a ½ cup serving: Less than 200 mg of Sodium

	CALORIES	SODIUM
Eden Foods Organic - No Salt Added		
Adzuki Beans	110	10
Black Beans	110	15
Black Eyed Peas	90	25
Cannellini Beans	100	40
Garbanzo Beans	130	30
Kidney Beans	100	15
Pinto Beans	110	15
Westbrae Organic		
Organic Black Beans	100	140
Great Northern Beans	100	140
Kidney Beans	100	140
Lentils	100	150
Pinto Beans	100	140
Red Beans	100	140

TOMATO/PASTA SAUCE
General Guidelines for a ½ cup serving: Less than 200 mg of Sodium

	CALORIES	SODIUM
Walnut Acres		
Low Sodium Tomato and Basil	40	20
Eden Foods		
No Salt Added Spaghetti Sauce	80	10
Enrico's		
Traditional with no salt	53	25
Millina's		
Organic Low Sodium Tomato and Basil	45	80
Francesco Rinaldi		
Grandma's Favorites, Traditional - no salt added	70	25

COMMERCIAL SEASONINGS

		CALORIES	SODIUM
Spike, no salt	*1 teaspoon*	0	0
VegeBase by Vogue	*1 teaspoon*	15	140
Mrs. Dash	*1 teaspoon*	0	0
Dr. Fuhrman's VegiZest	*1 teaspoon*	7	3
Nutritional Yeast	*1 tablespoon*	30	3

Note: This product has a nutty, cheesy flavor and can be used as an alternative to parmesan cheese.

Braggs Liquid Aminos	*1/2 teaspoon*	0	110

* Note: This is an all-purpose seasoning derived from soy beans and can be used as an alternative to soy sauce. It still contains the same amount of sodium as low-sodium soy sauce (600 mg per tablespoon) so limit your use to 1/2 teaspoon/serving.

Low Sodium Soy Sauce	*1/2 teaspoon*	2	100

RAW NUT BUTTERS

2 tablespoons

	CALORIES	SODIUM
Raw Cashew Butter	200	5
Raw Almond Butter	220	5

DR. FUHRMAN'S FLAVORED VINEGARS

1 tablespoon

	CALORIES	SODIUM
Spicy Pecan	5	0
Riesling Raisin	5	0
Blood Orange	5	0
Black Fig	5	0
D'Anjou Pear	5	0

All of the *Eat For Health* recipes are listed below. For easy reference, their MANDI Score is included along with the phase in which they were used. As you plan your own menus, use the MANDI scores to maximize the nutrient density of your diet. You can use recipes from any phase as long as you strive for a total daily score of 100.

SMOOTHIES, JUICES AND BLENDED SALADS

	PAGE	PHASE	MANDI SCORE
Blueberry Orange Smoothie	103	1	8.5
Chocolate Smoothie	104	3,4	19.0
Creamy Fruit and Berry Smoothie	105	2	12.5
Creamy Greeny Blended Salad	106	4	12.0
Eat Your Greens Fruit Smoothie	107	4	18.0
High Cruciferous Juice	108	4	27.5
Lisa's Favorite Green Smoothie	109	3	12.5
Mixed Vegetable Juice	110	4	35.5

BREAKFAST

	PAGE	PHASE	MANDI SCORE
Banana-Cashew Lettuce Wrap	111	3	6.0
Blueberry Nut Oatmeal	112	2	5.5
Cinnamon Fruit Oatmeal	113	1	7.0
Oatmeal and Fruit Compote	114	3	10.0
Pomegranate Muesli	115	2	10.0
Quick Banana Breakfast To Go	116	4	11.0
Special Oatmeal	117	3, 4	5.0

SALADS, DRESSINGS, AND DIPS

	PAGE	PHASE	MANDI SCORE
SALADS			
Asparagus Shiitake Salad with Creamy Sesame Dressing*	118	4	11.5
Balsamic Mixed Greens with Chopped Apples*	120	1	11.5
Citrus Salad with Orange Peanut Dressing	121	3	16.5
Crazy-About-Carrot Salad	122	3	13.5
Greek Chickpea Salad	123	4	9.0
Green Velvet Vegetable Salad	124	2	18.0
Greens and Berries Salad with Cashew Currant Dressing	125	3	23.0
Greens and Brown Rice with Pine Nuts, Apples, and Currants	126	4	10.0

Chocolate Dip	146	2	4.0
Creamy Sesame Dressing/Dip*	147	4	2.5
Dijon Date Dressing/Dip	148	2	2.5
Dijon Pistachio Dressing/Dip	149	3	2.0
Eggplant Hummus	150	2	6.5
Garbanzo Guacamole	151	1	9.0
Green Velvet Dressing/Dip	152	2	4.0
Hot Pepper Salsa	153	1	2.5
Orange Cashew Dressing/Dip	154	2	3.0
Orange Peanut Dressing/Dip	155	3	1.5
Red Pepper Salsa*	156	2	4.0
Russian Fig Dressing/Dip	157	1, 4	2.5
Sesame Fig Dressing/Dip*	158	2	2.5
Spicy Bean Spread/Dip	159	4	3.0
Strawberry Dressing/Sauce	160	3	3.5
Tahini Dressing/Dip	161	3	3.0
Tasty Hummus	162	1,2	3.0
Tofu Ranch Dressing/Dip	163	2, 4	1.5
Tomato Almond Dressing/Dip	164	3	3.5

SOUPS AND STEWS

	PAGE	PHASE	MANDI SCORE
Black Forest Cream of Mushroom Soup	165	3	19.0
Chunky Sweet Potato Stew*	167	1	13.5
Dr. Fuhrman's Famous Anti-Cancer Soup	168	3	29.5
Fast Black Bean Soup	170	1	20.0
French Minted Pea Soup	171	4	9.0
Gazpacho Summer Soup	172	2	21.0
Hearty Ginger Lentil Soup	173	2	26.0
Hearty Vegetable Stew	175	4	36.0
High Cruciferous Vegetable Stew	177	4	34.0
Quick and Creamy Vegetable Bean Soup	179	2	22.0
Speedy Vegetable and Bean Soup	180	3	28.0
Tomato Bean Barley Soup*	181	1	11.0
West African Lentil Okra Stew	182	2	30.5

NON-VEGAN DISHES

Limit animal products to eight servings/week in Phase One; five servings/week in Phase Two; three servings/week in Phase Three; and two servings/week in Phase Four.

	PAGE	PHASE	MANDI SCORE
Creole Chicken with Spinach and Rice	183	2	13.5
Dijon Chicken	185	1	2.5
Egg and Vegetable Scramble	186	3	21.0
Filet of Sole with Mango Salsa	187	4	3.5
Garden Eggs and Tofu with Salsa	188	4	12.5
Pasta with Shrimp and Artichokes*	190	3	8.0
Salsa Salmon over Wilted Greens	192	2	14.0

VEGAN DISHES

DESSERTS

	PAGE	PHASE	MANDI SCORE
Apple Surprise	253	4	5.5
Banana Fig Ice Cream	254	3	2.0
Banana Pumpkin Pudding	255	2	11.5
Banana Walnut Ice Cream	256	2	2.5
Berry Cobbler	257	4	3.5
Bluevado Pie	258	3	4.5
Frozen Banana Fluff	259	1	2.5
Fruit and Berry Compote	260	2	8.5
Fruit and Nut Bowl	261	2	10.0
Healthy Chocolate Cake	262	4	9.0
Jenna's Peach Freeze	264	1	3.5
Macadamia Cream	265	1	1.5
Mango Riesling Compote	266	1	4.5
Mixed Berry Freeze	267	3	8.5
Nutrient-Rich Chocolate Pudding	268	3	13.0
Poached Pears with Raspberry Sauce	270	1	4.5
Strawberry Pineapple Sorbet	271	4	9.0
Very Berry Ice Cream	272	1	6.5
Wild Apple Crunch	273	1	3.5
Yummy Banana-Oat Bars	274	2	2.5

Contains olive oil or sesame oil. Limit to one tablespoon/day in Phases One and Two, and two tablespoons/week in Phase Three. Use minimal amounts in Phase Four.

BLUEBERRY ORANGE SMOOTHIE

MANDI
8.5

Serves: 2 — Prep Time: 5 minutes

INGREDIENTS

3 dates, pitted

2 oranges, peeled

1 banana

1 cup frozen blueberries

1 tablespoon ground flax seeds

DIRECTIONS

Blend all ingredients together in a high powered blender until smooth and creamy.

One Serving Contains:
CALORIES 207.4; PROTEIN 2.3g; CARBOHYDRATE 48.7g; FAT 2.4g; SODIUM 2.7mg

CHOCOLATE SMOOTHIE

MANDI
19

Serves: 2 — Prep Time: 5 minutes

INGREDIENTS

5 ounces organic baby spinach

2 cups frozen blueberries

1/2 cup soy milk

1 medium banana

2 medjool dates or 4 deglet noor dates

2 tablespoons *Dr. Fuhrman's Cocoa Powder*
or other natural cocoa powder

1 tablespoon ground flax seeds

DIRECTIONS

Blend all ingredients together in a high powered blender until smooth and creamy.

One Serving Contains:
CALORIES 276.2; PROTEIN 8.1g; CARBOHYDRATE 58.8g; FAT 4.8g; SODIUM 93.4mg

CREAMY FRUIT AND BERRY SMOOTHIE

MANDI
12.5

Serves: 2 — Prep Time: 6 minutes

INGREDIENTS

1 cup pomegranate juice

1/2 cup soy or almond milk

1/2 cup frozen strawberries

1/2 cup frozen blueberries

1/2 cup frozen peaches

1 banana

1 tablespoon ground flax seeds

DIRECTIONS

Blend all ingredients together in a high powered blender.

One Serving Contains:
CALORIES 225; PROTEIN 4.9g; CARBOHYDRATE 47.7g; FAT 3.2g; SODIUM 40.8mg

CREAMY GREENY BLENDED SALAD

MANDI
12

Serves: 2 — Prep Time: 5 minutes

INGREDIENTS

4 ounces (4 cups) organic baby spinach

4 cups torn romaine lettuce

1/4 cup pecan halves

1/3 cup soy milk

4 medjool dates, pitted (or 7 regular pitted dates)

DIRECTIONS

Blend all ingredients together in a high powered blender and blend until smooth and creamy.

One Serving Contains:
CALORIES 280.0; PROTEIN 6.9g; CARBOHYDRATE 45.6g; FAT 11.2g; SODIUM 76.2mg

EAT YOUR GREENS FRUIT SMOOTHIE

MANDI
18

Serves: 2 — Prep Time: 3 minutes

INGREDIENTS

5 ounces organic baby spinach

1 medium banana

1 cup frozen or fresh blueberries

1/2 cup soy milk

1/2 cup pomegranate juice or other unsweetened fruit juice

1 tablespoon ground flax seeds

DIRECTIONS

Blend all ingredients together in a high powered blender
until smooth and creamy.

One Serving Contains:
CALORIES 195.7; PROTEIN 6.4g; CARBOHYDRATE 38.7g; FAT 3.6g; SODIUM 93.9mg

HIGH CRUCIFEROUS JUICE

MANDI 27.5

Serves: 4 — Prep Time: 20 minutes

INGREDIENTS

6 medium carrots

6 cauliflower florets

2 apples, cut in fourths

1 bunch kale

1/2 bunch watercress

1/2 head broccoli with stems

DIRECTIONS

Run all ingredients through a juicer.

One Serving Contains:
CALORIES 128.2; PROTEIN 7.4g; CARBOHYDRATE 29g; FAT 0.9g; SODIUM 121.6mg

LISA'S FAVORITE GREEN SMOOTHIE

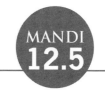

Serves: 2 — Prep Time: 5 minutes

INGREDIENTS

1 apple*, cut into fourths

1 banana

1/2 avocado

4 pitted dates (or 3 *Dr. Fuhrman's Original Date Nut Pop'ems*)

5 ounces organic baby spinach

DIRECTIONS

Blend all ingredients in a high powered blender
until smooth and creamy.

*No need to peel apple if organic.

One Serving Contains:
CALORIES 242.7; PROTEIN 6.5g; CARBOHYDRATE 44g; FAT 8.3g; SODIUM 59.1mg

MIXED VEGETABLE JUICE

MANDI
21

Serves: 3 — Prep Time: 20 minutes

INGREDIENTS

6 kale leaves

8 carrots, peeled

2 stalks bok choy

2 apples

2 medium beets, peeled

1 cup watercress with stems

DIRECTIONS

Run all ingredients through a juicer.

One Serving Contains:
CALORIES 157.3; PROTEIN 7.1g; CARBOHYDRATE 36.6g; FAT 0.9g; SODIUM 181.1mg

BANANA - CASHEW LETTUCE WRAP

MANDI
6

Serves: 2 — Prep Time: 5 minutes

INGREDIENTS

4 tablespoons raw cashew butter

12 romaine lettuce leaves

2 bananas, thinly sliced

DIRECTIONS

Spread cashew butter on lettuce leaf (1 teaspoon per leaf)

Lay banana slices on cashew butter and wrap lettuce around.

One Serving Contains:
CALORIES 311.9; PROTEIN 8.3g; CARBOHYDRATE 39.5g; FAT 16.5g; SODIUM 14.9mg

THIS MAKES
A DELICIOUS,
HEALTHY
BREAKFAST
OR SNACK.

BLUEBERRY NUT OATMEAL

MANDI
5.5

Serves: 3 — Prep Time: 8 minutes

INGREDIENTS

1 3/4 cups water

1 cup old fashioned rolled oats

1 cup grated apple

2 tablespoons currants (optional)

1 tablespoon ground flax seeds

1 cup fresh or frozen blueberries

6 pecan halves, chopped

DIRECTIONS

In a saucepan, bring water to a boil and stir in all ingredients, except blueberries and pecans. Turn heat down and simmer for 5 minutes.

Stir in blueberries and pecans. Remove from heat and cover for 2-3 minutes before serving.

One Serving Contains:
CALORIES 185.1; PROTEIN 11.5g; CARBOHYDRATE 31.9g; FAT 5.9g; SODIUM 5.7mg

Cinnamon Fruit Oatmeal

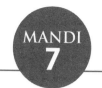

MANDI
7

Serves: 2 — Prep Time: 15 minutes

INGREDIENTS

1 cup water

1 teaspoon vanilla extract

1/4 teaspoon cinnamon

1/2 cup old-fashioned rolled oats

1/2 cup blueberries

2 apples, chopped

2 tablespoons chopped walnuts

1 tablespoon ground flax seeds

1/4 cup raisins (optional)

DIRECTIONS

In a saucepan, combine water with the vanilla and cinnamon. Bring to a boil over high heat. Reduce the heat to a simmer and stir in the oats.

When the mixture starts to simmer, add the blueberries. Remove from heat when berries are heated through.

Cover and let stand for 15 minutes until thick and creamy.

Mix in apples, nuts, flax seeds, and raisins (if desired).

One Serving Contains:
CALORIES 240.7; PROTEIN 12.7g; CARBOHYDRATE 40.8g; FAT 8.1g; SODIUM 6.8mg

OATMEAL AND FRUIT COMPOTE

MANDI
10

Serves: 2 — Prep Time: 15 minutes

INGREDIENTS

fresh fruits, chopped

raisins or other dried fruits, chopped

soy milk, orange juice or pomegranate juice, to cover for soaking

1 cup old fashioned rolled oats

DIRECTIONS

To make fruit compote: Combine the fresh and dried fruits in a glass jar along with some soy milk or juice for soaking. Cover and refrigerate overnight.

In the morning, prepare rolled oats according to directions on package.

Add fruit compote to the oatmeal.

One Serving Contains:
CALORIES 245.2; PROTEIN 10.2g; CARBOHYDRATE 51.5g; FAT 3.3g; SODIUM 4.1mg

POMEGRANATE MUESLI

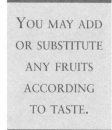

MANDI
10

Serves: 2 — Prep Time: 20 minutes

INGREDIENTS

1/2 cup pomegranate juice

1/4 cup oats, steel cut or old fashioned (not quick or instant)

1 apple, peeled and grated

4 raw cashews or hazelnuts, coarsely chopped

1/2 cup halved grapes

1/2 cup cubed cantaloupe

1/2 cup sliced fresh organic strawberries

1 tablespoon currants (optional)

1 tablespoon ground flax seeds

> YOU MAY ADD OR SUBSTITUTE ANY FRUITS ACCORDING TO TASTE.

DIRECTIONS

Soak oats in pomegranate juice overnight in refrigerator. Oats will absorb the liquid.

In the morning, combine oats with remaining ingredients.

One Serving Contains:
CALORIES 258.2; PROTEIN 7.2g; CARBOHYDRATE 43.6g; FAT 8.7g; SODIUM 13.4mg

QUICK BANANA BREAKFAST TO GO

Serves: 2 — Prep Time: 8 minutes

INGREDIENTS

2 cups frozen blueberries

1/2 cup old-fashioned rolled oats

1/3 cup pomegranate juice

2 tablespoons dried currants (optional)

2 tablespoons chopped walnuts

1 tablespoon raw sunflower seeds

2 bananas, sliced

DIRECTIONS

In cereal bowl, combine all ingredients.

Heat in microwave for 3 minutes.

One Serving Contains:
CALORIES 357.5; PROTEIN 6.7g; CARBOHYDRATE 67.3g; FAT 9.9g; SODIUM 4.7mg

ON THE GO, COMBINE ALL INGREDIENTS IN A SEALED CONTAINER AND EAT LATER, EITHER HOT OR COLD.

SPECIAL OATMEAL

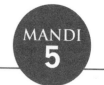

Serves: 4 — Prep Time: 20 minutes

INGREDIENTS

1 3/4 cups water

1 cup old-fashioned rolled oats

6 pitted dates, chopped

1/4 teaspoon coriander

2 bananas, sliced

1 cup chopped or grated apple

1 cup frozen or fresh blueberries

1 tablespoon ground flax seeds

DIRECTIONS

In saucepan, bring water to a boil and stir in all ingredients, except blueberries and flax seeds. Simmer for 5 minutes.

Stir in blueberries. Sprinkle flax seeds on top or stir in. Cover for 2-3 minutes before serving.

One Serving Contains:
CALORIES 206.9; PROTEIN 9.3g; CARBOHYDRATE 46.4g; FAT 2.6g; SODIUM 5.1mg

IF DESIRED, THIS RECIPE MAY BE MADE IN THE OVEN. PREHEAT OVEN TO 350 DEGREES. IN A BAKING DISH, COMBINE ALL INGREDIENTS, EXCEPT FOR THE BANANAS, APPLES, BLUEBERRIES, AND FLAX SEEDS. BAKE UNCOVERED FOR 30 MINUTES. ADD THE BANANA AND MORE WATER, IF DESIRED. BAKE ANOTHER 15 MINUTES. STIR IN APPLE AND BLUEBERRIES. SPRINKLE FLAX SEEDS ON TOP.

SALADS

ASPARAGUS SHIITAKE SALAD WITH CREAMY SESAME DRESSING

MANDI
11.5

Serves: 4 — Prep Time: 30 minutes

INGREDIENTS - CREAMY SESAME DRESSING

1 cup soy milk

2/3 cup unhulled sesame seeds, lightly toasted*

2 tablespoons *Dr. Fuhrman's Riesling Raisin Vinegar*
  or seasoned rice vinegar

1 tablespoon raw cashew butter

1 teaspoon toasted sesame oil

7 pitted dates, or to taste, soaked in water 30 minutes
  (reserve soaking water)

1/2 clove garlic

2 tablespoons unhulled sesame seeds, lightly toasted*

INGREDIENTS - SALAD

2 medium beets, peeled and sliced 1/2 inch thick

1/2 pound shiitake mushrooms, sliced

1 pound fresh asparagus, cut diagonally into 2 inch slices

1 tablespoon *Dr. Fuhrman's VegiZest*
  or other no salt soup base seasoning

1 teaspoon garlic powder

continued...

ASPARAGUS SHIITAKE SALAD WITH
CREAMY SESAME DRESSING *continued...*

1 red bell pepper, seeded and thinly sliced

1/2 cup sliced water chestnuts

4 cups watercress

2 cups bean sprouts

DIRECTIONS

In a high powered blender, blend all dressing ingredients, except for the 2 tablespoons sesame seeds, until smooth and creamy. Stir in remaining sesame seeds. Use soaking water from dates to thin if needed.

Preheat oven to 400 degrees.

Place beets in a baking pan and add 1/2 cup water. Cover and roast for 20 minutes. Uncover and continue roasting until tender. If needed, add more water to keep beets from drying out. Set aside.

Meanwhile, water sauté mushrooms over high heat for about 7 minutes, using only enough water to keep from scorching. When mushrooms are tender and juicy add asparagus and water sauté until slightly tender, but still crisp. Toss in VegiZest and garlic powder. Remove from heat and toss with bell pepper and water chestnuts.

Place watercress on plate and pile vegetable mixture on top.

Drizzle dressing over all and top with bean sprouts.

Arrange roasted beets around the sides.

*Lightly toast sesame seeds in a pan over medium heat for three minutes, shaking pan frequently.

One Serving Contains:
CALORIES 225.9; PROTEIN 12.1g; CARBOHYDRATE 35g; FAT 7g; SODIUM 107.6mg

BALSAMIC MIXED GREENS WITH CHOPPED APPLES

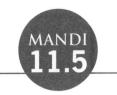

MANDI
11.5

Serves: 2 — Prep Time: 15 minutes

INGREDIENTS - QUICK BALSAMIC VINAIGRETTE

4 tablespoons balsamic vinegar

2 tablespoons fig preserves

2 tablespoons olive oil

INGREDIENTS - SALAD

1 head (about 6 cups) romaine lettuce, torn in bite-sized pieces

4 ounces or 4 cups baby salad mix

2 apples, chopped

1/2 cup fresh raspberries (optional)

DIRECTIONS

Whisk all dressing ingredients together using a fork or wire whisk.

Mix greens, add fruit, and then toss with dressing.

Low fat, low salt bottled dressing may be substituted for the balsamic vinaigrette.

One Serving Contains:
CALORIES 329.2; PROTEIN 6.9g; CARBOHYDRATE 48.3g; FAT 14.5g; SODIUM 41.5mg

Citrus Salad
with Orange Peanut Dressing

MANDI
16.5

Serves: 2 — Prep Time: 15 minutes

INGREDIENTS - ORANGE PEANUT DRESSING

1/2 cup orange juice

2 tablespoons peanut butter, unsalted

2 tablespoons raw cashew butter

2 tablespoons rice vinegar

1 teaspoon Bragg Liquid Aminos
or low sodium soy sauce

1/4 inch piece fresh ginger, peeled

1/4 medium clove garlic, chopped

Dressing yields
four servings.
Leftover dressing
may be stored in
the refrigerator
for 2 to 3 days.

INGREDIENTS - SALAD

15 ounces or 10 cups baby lettuce mix

1 avocado, sliced

1 orange, peeled, cut in half and sliced

1/2 small sweet onion, thinly sliced and cut in half

1 tablespoon unhulled sesame seeds, lightly toasted*

DIRECTIONS

Blend all dressing ingredients in high powered blender or food processor
until smooth.

To prepare salad, arrange avocado slices, onions, and orange rounds on
top of lettuce. Pour dressing over salad and sprinkle with sesame seeds.

Lightly toast sesame seeds in a pan over medium heat for three minutes, shaking pan frequently.

One Serving Contains:
CALORIES 408.6; PROTEIN 11.8g; CARBOHYDRATE 40.0g; FAT 26.3g; SODIUM 91.8mg

CRAZY ABOUT CARROT SALAD

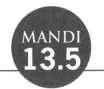

Serves: 2 — Prep Time: 8 minutes

INGREDIENTS

8 medium carrots, shredded

1/2 cup raisins

4 tablespoons fresh orange juice

1/4 teaspoon cinnamon, or to taste

DIRECTIONS

Combine carrots and raisins.

Add orange juice and cinnamon and mix all ingredients together.

One Serving Contains:
CALORIES 223.1; PROTEIN 3.5g; CARBOHYDRATE 55.5g; FAT 0.8g; SODIUM 172.7mg

GREEK CHICKPEA SALAD

MANDI
9

Serves: 4 — Prep Time: 25 minutes

INGREDIENTS

1 16-ounce can garbanzo beans (chick peas), no or low salt

3 plum tomatoes, chopped

1 boiled potato, peeled and chopped in chunks

1 green apple, peeled, cored and chopped

1 cucumber, chopped

1/2 small onion, chopped

2 tablespoons chopped brazil nuts, (optional)

3 tablespoons *Dr. Fuhrman's Spicy Pecan Vinegar*

1 teaspoon chopped cilantro

10 ounces mixed salad greens

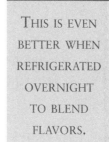

THIS IS EVEN BETTER WHEN REFRIGERATED OVERNIGHT TO BLEND FLAVORS.

DIRECTIONS

Mix all ingredients, except salad greens. Serve on bed of mixed salad greens.

One Serving Contains:
CALORIES 288.1; PROTEIN 15.3g; CARBOHYDRATE 54.2g; FAT 3.5g; SODIUM 22.9mg

GREEN VELVET VEGETABLE SALAD

MANDI
18

Serves: 2 — Prep Time: 25 minutes

INGREDIENTS - GREEN VELVET DRESSING

3/4 cup water

1/2 cup fresh lemon juice

1/2 cup raw tahini (pureed sesame seeds)

1/4 cup chopped fresh parsley

1/4 cup chopped fresh dill

4 tablespoons raw cashews

2 tablespoons *Dr. Fuhrman's VegiZest*

1/2 tablespoon chopped fresh tarragon (optional)

2 teaspoons Bragg Liquid Aminos or low sodium soy sauce

2 cloves garlic, chopped

> DRESSING YIELDS FOUR SERVINGS. LEFTOVER DRESSING MAY BE STORED IN THE REFRIGERATOR FOR 2 TO 3 DAYS.

INGREDIENTS - SALAD

10 ounces (about 10 cups) mixed salad greens

1/2 cup shredded zucchini

1/2 cup fresh or frozen corn

1/2 cup diced red bell pepper

1/4 cup chopped scallions

1 cup sprouts (assorted varieties)

DIRECTIONS

Blend all dressing ingredients in a high powered blender until smooth.

Toss salad ingredients with dressing and top with sprouts..

One Serving Contains:
CALORIES 346.9; PROTEIN 14.8g; CARBOHYDRATE 38.2g; FAT 19.7g; SODIUM 199.4mg

GREENS AND BERRIES SALAD
WITH CASHEW CURRANT DRESSING

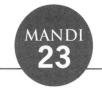

Serves: 2 — Prep Time: 15 minutes

INGREDIENTS - CASHEW CURRANT DRESSING

1/4 cup raw cashews or 2 ounces raw cashew butter

1/3 cup soy milk

1/4 cup unsweetened applesauce

2 tablespoons dried currants or raisins

INGREDIENTS - SALAD

1 head (about 6 cups) romaine lettuce

5 ounces (about 5 cups) organic baby spinach

1 12-ounce bag frozen strawberries, defrosted and sliced in half

DIRECTIONS

To make dressing, blend cashews or cashew butter with soy milk and applesauce in a high powered blender until smooth. Add the currants and blend well.

Pile the lettuce and spinach leaves on a plate and lay the strawberries on top. Pour the juice from the strawberries over the greens.

Drizzle dressing over the greens and berries.

One Serving Contains:
CALORIES 351.6; PROTEIN 12.7g; CARBOHYDRATE 44.5g; FAT 17.6g; SODIUM 101.0mg

GREENS AND BROWN RICE SALAD WITH PINE NUTS, APPLES, AND CURRANTS

MANDI
10

Serves: 2 — Prep Time: 10 minutes

INGREDIENTS

1/2 cup cooked brown rice

10 ounces (about 10 cups) baby greens

1 apple, peeled & grated

1/2 cup currants

5 tablespoons balsamic vinegar

2 tablespoons *Dr. Fuhrman's Riesling Raisin Vinegar*

1/4 cup pine nuts

DIRECTIONS

Cook rice according to package directions.

Toss all ingredients except pine nuts.

Sprinkle with pine nuts and serve.

One Serving Contains:
CALORIES 381.2; PROTEIN 8.8g; CARBOHYDRATE 64.1g; FAT 12.8g; SODIUM 28.6mg

GREENS AND VEGETABLES WITH SESAME FIG DRESSING

MANDI
19

Serves: 2 — Prep Time: 15 minutes

INGREDIENTS - SESAME FIG DRESSING

1/4 cup water

1/4 cup raw tahini

2 tablespoons fig preserves

1 tablespoon sesame oil

1 tablespoon *Dr. Fuhrman's Black Fig Vinegar*

INGREDIENTS - SALAD

4 ounces (about 4 cups) mixed baby greens

1 head (about 6 cups) romaine lettuce

2 carrots, grated

1 green pepper, chopped

1/2 pint cherry tomatoes

> DRESSING YIELDS
> 4 SERVINGS.
> LEFTOVER
> DRESSING MAY BE
> STORED IN THE
> REFRIGERATOR
> FOR 2-3 DAYS.

DIRECTIONS

Using wire whisk or blender, blend dressing ingredients until smooth and creamy.

Toss greens and vegetables with dressing.

One Serving Contains:
CALORIES 250.8; PROTEIN 11.3g; CARBOHYDRATE 33.4g; FAT 11.8g; SODIUM 92.9mg

HEALTHY SLAW

MANDI
9.5

Serves: 3 — Prep Time: 20 minutes

INGREDIENTS - SLAW

2 cups shredded apples

1 cup shredded raw cabbage

1 cup shredded raw beets

1 cup shredded raw carrots

1/2 cup raisins

INGREDIENTS - DRESSING

1/2 cup soft tofu

1/4 cup soy milk

1 tablespoon *Dr. Fuhrman's Riesling Raisin Vinegar*

1 tablespoon *Dr. Fuhrman's Spicy Pecan Vinegar*

1 tablespoon date sugar

2 teaspoons fresh lemon juice

1/4 cup chopped pecans, lightly toasted*(optional)

DIRECTIONS

Combine slaw ingredients.

Blend dressing ingredients and toss with slaw.

If desired, sprinkle toasted pecans over slaw.

Lightly toast pecans in a 200 degree oven for 3 minutes.

One Serving Contains:
CALORIES 201; PROTEIN 5.5g; CARBOHYDRATE 47.5g; FAT 1.2g; SODIUM 83mg

INDIAN MANGO SALAD

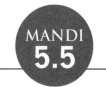

Serves: 4 — Prep Time: 10 minutes

INGREDIENTS

2 organic celery stalks, chopped

2 ripe mangos, peeled and sliced

2 firm tomatoes, chopped

1 red bell pepper, chopped

1 small red onion, chopped

1/2 tablespoon *Dr. Fuhrman's VegiZest*

1 pinch chili powder

DIRECTIONS

Combine all ingredients in a bowl. Cover and refrigerate for 1 hour before serving to allow flavors to blend.

One Serving Contains:
CALORIES 118.3; PROTEIN 3.9g; CARBOHYDRATE 29.1g; FAT 0.6g; SODIUM 34mg

MISHMASH SALAD
WITH ORANGE CASHEW DRESSING

MANDI
23

Serves: 2 — Prep Time: 25 minutes

INGREDIENTS - ORANGE CASHEW DRESSING

2 oranges, peeled and seeded

1/4 cup raw cashews

2 tablespoons *Dr. Fuhrman's Blood Orange Vinegar*

2 carrots, grated

orange juice (optional)

INGREDIENTS - SALAD

1 head (about 6 cups) romaine lettuce

4 ounces (about 4 -6 cups) mixed greens

1 cup mache or watercress

1 cup orange sections

1 cup sliced fresh organic strawberries

1/4 cup dried apricots, coarsely chopped or Goji berries (optional)

2 tablespoons unhulled sesame seeds, lightly toasted* (optional)

DIRECTIONS

Blend dressing ingredients in a high powered blender until smooth and creamy. Add some orange juice to thin dressing, if necessary.

Combine salad ingredients

Toss dressing with salad. If desired, sprinkle with sesame seeds.

Lightly toast sesame seeds in a pan over medium heat for three minutes, shaking pan frequently.

One Serving Contains:
CALORIES 329.6; PROTEIN 8.8g; CARBOHYDRATE 60.5g; FAT 8.9g; SODIUM 77.3mg

MIXED GREENS AND FRUIT WITH BLUEBERRY DRESSING

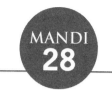

MANDI
28

Serves: 2 — Prep Time: 30 minutes

INGREDIENTS - BLUEBERRY DRESSING

2 cups fresh or frozen blueberries, thawed

1/4 cup unhulled sesame seeds

1/4 cup sunflower seeds

1/2 cup pomegranate juice

4 tablespoons *Dr. Fuhrman's Wild Blueberry Vinegar*

INGREDIENTS - SALAD

2 heads (about 12 cups) romaine lettuce, washed & torn into bite-sized pieces

2 kiwis, cut into pieces

1 pint fresh organic strawberries, halved

1 apple, cut into chunks

1 pear, cut into chunks

2 ounces chopped pecans (optional)

DRESSING YIELDS 4 SERVINGS. LEFTOVER DRESSING MAY BE STORED IN THE REFRIGERATOR FOR 2-3 DAYS.

ANY COMBINATION OF THESE FRUITS MAY BE USED OR OTHER FRUITS MAY BE SUBSTITUTED IN THIS SALAD.

DIRECTIONS

Puree all dressing ingredients in a high powered blender until smooth.

Toss salad ingredients together.

Combine dressing and salad. Sprinkle with chopped pecans if desired.

One Serving Contains:
CALORIES 397.6; PROTEIN 12.1g; CARBOHYDRATE 73.5g; FAT 11.5g; SODIUM 36.6mg

ORANGE SESAME TOSSED SALAD

MANDI
17

Serves: 2 — Prep Time: 15 minutes

INGREDIENTS

> 3 tablespoons unhulled sesame seeds, toasted*, divided
>
> 12 raw cashew nuts
>
> 1/2 cup orange juice
>
> 2 tablespoons *Dr. Fuhrman's Riesling Raisin Vinegar*
> or seasoned rice vinegar
>
> 2 oranges, peeled and diced,
> or 1 jar unsweetened mandarin orange slices
>
> 2 heads (12 cups) romaine lettuce, torn in bite-sized pieces

DIRECTIONS

> In a high powered blender, blend 2 tablespoons sesame seeds, cashews, orange juice, and vinegar until creamy and smooth. Add additional orange juice to thin if necessary.
>
> Combine diced oranges with romaine lettuce and toss with dressing.
>
> Sprinkle the remaining sesame seeds on top.

*Lightly toast the sesame seeds in a pan over medium heat for 3 minutes, shaking the pan frequently.

One Serving Contains:
CALORIES 383.9; PROTEIN 12.5g; CARBOHYDRATE 44.8g; FAT 20.4g; SODIUM 33.1mg

QUINOA BEAN SALAD

MANDI
8

Serves: 6 — Prep Time: 25 minutes

INGREDIENTS

2 cups cooked quinoa

1 15-ounce can white beans (low or no salt), drained

1 cup grated carrots

1 cup currants

1/2 cup raw walnuts, chopped

2 plum tomatoes, chopped

1 small red onion, thinly sliced

1/2 green pepper, chopped

1/2 red pepper, chopped

1/2 orange or yellow pepper, chopped

3 cloves garlic, minced

1 tablespoon chili powder

2 teaspoons Bragg Liquid Aminos or low sodium soy sauce

1/2 cup Goji berries (optional)

THE VEGETABLES MAY BE CHOPPED IN A FOOD PROCESSOR TO SAVE TIME.

THIS IS EVEN BETTER WHEN REFRIGERATED OVERNIGHT TO BLEND FLAVORS.

DIRECTIONS

Cook quinoa according to package directions.

Place all other ingredients in a large bowl and mix.

Add cooked quinoa and toss.

One Serving Contains:
CALORIES 383.2; PROTEIN 14.6g; CARBOHYDRATE 67g; FAT 9g; SODIUM 122.3mg

RAISIN COLESLAW

MANDI
9

Serves: 6 — Prep Time: 20 minutes

INGREDIENTS

1/2 cup raisins

1/2 cup apple juice

1/2 cup baked potato, skin removed

1 teaspoon mustard

1 tablespoon lemon juice

4 cups shredded cabbage

2 cups shredded carrots

2 cups peeled and shredded apples

1 cup shredded beets (optional)

1/4 cup finely chopped scallions

> USE THIS IN PLACE
> OF A LETTUCE
> SALAD FOR LUNCH
> OR DINNER.

DIRECTIONS

Blend the raisins, apple juice, potato, mustard, and lemon juice in a high powered blender.

Mix with remaining ingredients.

One Serving Contains:
CALORIES 119.5; PROTEIN 3.6g; CARBOHYDRATE 29.6g; FAT 0.4g; SODIUM 65.8mg

ROMAINE, SPINACH, WATERCRESS SALAD WITH FRUIT AND NUTS

MANDI 20

Serves: 2 — Prep Time: 20 minutes

INGREDIENTS - BALSAMIC VINAIGRETTE

1/2 cup water

6 tablespoons roasted garlic rice vinegar

4 tablespoons olive oil

4 tablespoons balsamic vinegar

4 tablespoons 100% grape fruit spread or raisins

4 cloves garlic, pressed

1 teaspoon dried oregano

1/2 teaspoon dried basil

1/2 teaspoon onion powder

> VINAIGRETTE YIELDS 1 1/3 CUPS. STORE LEFTOVER DRESSING IN THE REFRIGERATOR FOR UP TO ONE WEEK.
>
> A LOW FAT, LOW SALT BOTTLED BALSAMIC VINAIGRETTE MAY ALSO BE USED.

INGREDIENTS - SALAD

1 head (about 6 cups) romaine lettuce, shredded

5 ounces (about 5 cups) organic baby spinach

1/2 bunch watercress leaves

1 apple, grated

1 pear, grated

4 tablespoons chopped walnuts

1/4 cup raisins or currents (optional)

DIRECTIONS

Blend all vinaigrette ingredients together in a high powered blender.

Combine salad ingredients. Toss salad with light amount of vinaigrette.

One Serving Contains:
CALORIES 228.3; PROTEIN 9.2g; CARBOHYDRATE 32.9g; FAT 10.6g; SODIUM 85.2mg

SOUTHERN-STYLE MIXED GREENS

MANDI
14

Serves: 2 — Prep Time: 15 minutes

INGREDIENTS

1 cup water

1 clove garlic, minced

dash of black pepper

1 15-ounce can black eyed peas (no or low salt)*, rinsed and drained

1 cup chopped yellow peppers

1 cup chopped tomato

1/3 cup chopped fresh parsley

1/4 cup chopped red onion

1/8 cup balsamic vinegar or low fat dressing

10 ounces (about 7 cups) mixed salad greens

DIRECTIONS

Combine water, garlic, and black pepper in a large saucepan; bring to a boil. Add black eyed peas; cover and simmer over low heat for 10 minutes. Drain.

In a bowl, combine black eyed peas with yellow peppers and next four ingredients. Cover and chill for 3 hours or overnight.

Serve over salad greens.

If you can't find low or no salt black eyed peas, use low or no salt small white beans instead.

One Serving Contains:
CALORIES 390.4; PROTEIN 24.6g; CARBOHYDRATE 73.9g; FAT 2.1g; SODIUM 39.4mg

SUNSHINE SLAW

MANDI
7.5

Serves: 4 — Prep Time: 8 minutes

INGREDIENTS

4 carrots, grated

1 1/2 apples, peeled and chopped

1 teaspoon fresh lemon juice

1/3 cup raisins

1/3 cup slivered or sliced almonds

1/3 cup low salt mayonnaise or Vegenaise (a vegan alternative)

DIRECTIONS

Toss carrots and apples with lemon juice. Add raisins and almonds.

Mix in low salt mayonnaise or Vegenaise.

One Serving Contains:
CALORIES 183.5; PROTEIN 3.5g; CARBOHYDRATE 27.4g; FAT 8.4g; SODIUM 64.6mg

TOSSED SALAD
WITH DIJON PISTACHIO DRESSING

MANDI
12.5

Serves: 2 — Prep Time: 20 minutes

INGREDIENTS - DIJON PISTACHIO DRESSING

2/3 cup water

1/2 cup pistachio nuts, unsalted, preferably raw

2 tablespoons lemon juice

1 tablespoon ground flax seeds

2 teaspoons *Dr. Fuhrman's VegiZest*

1 teaspoon Dijon mustard

1/2 teaspoon Bragg Liquid Aminos or low sodium soy sauce

1/4 teaspoon garlic powder

2 deglet noor dates or 1 medjool date (optional)

INGREDIENTS - SALAD

10 ounces (about 10 cups) mixed greens

1 medium tomato, chopped or handful of cherry tomatoes, halved

1 carrot, grated

1/2 medium cucumber, halved and thinly sliced

1/2 small red onion, chopped

DIRECTIONS

Blend dressing ingredients in high powered blender until smooth and creamy.

Combine salad ingredients and toss with dressing.

One Serving Contains:
CALORIES 318; PROTEIN 13.8g; CARBOHYDRATE 37.7g; FAT 16.4g; SODIUM 181.7mg

Tropical Fruit Salad

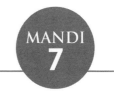

Serves: 4 — Prep Time: 20 minutes

INGREDIENTS

2 cups cubed pineapple

1 cup cubed mango

1 cup cubed papaya

2 oranges, peeled and sliced

1 banana, sliced

2 tablespoons unsweetened shredded coconut

shredded romaine lettuce, optional

DIRECTIONS

Toss fruit together. Add coconut and serve on top of lettuce, if desired.
Serve immediately.

One Serving Contains:
CALORIES 145.9; PROTEIN 1.6g; CARBOHYDRATE 35.5g; FAT 1.3g; SODIUM 4.6mg

WALNUT-PEAR GREEN SALAD

MANDI
10

Serves: 2 — Prep Time: 10 minutes

INGREDIENTS

8 ounces (about 8 cups) baby salad mix

2 ounces (about 2 cups) arugula or watercress

1 pear, grated

1/4 cup currants

1/4 cup walnuts, crushed or chopped

2 tablespoons *Dr. Fuhrman's D'Anjou Pear Vinegar*
   or balsamic vinegar

2 teaspoons olive oil

2 pears, peeled and sliced

1/4 cup walnut halves (optional)

> USE WATERCRESS AS
> OFTEN AS POSSIBLE
> IN SALADS FOR
> NUTRIENT DENSITY.

DIRECTIONS

Combine greens with grated pear, currants, and walnuts. Toss with vinegar & olive oil.

Top with sliced pears and if desired, walnut halves.

One Serving Contains:
CALORIES 145.9; PROTEIN 1.6g; CARBOHYDRATE 35.5g; FAT 1.3g; SODIUM 4.6mg

SALADS, DRESSINGS AND DIPS

DRESSINGS AND DIPS

BALSAMIC VINAIGRETTE

Serves: 5 — Prep Time: 8 minutes

INGREDIENTS

1/2 cup water

6 tablespoons roasted garlic rice vinegar

4 tablespoons olive oil

4 tablespoons balsamic vinegar

4 tablespoons 100% grape fruit spread or raisins

4 cloves garlic, pressed

1 teaspoon dried oregano

1/2 teaspoon dried basil

1/2 teaspoon onion powder

DIRECTIONS

Blend all ingredients together in a high powered blender.

Yields: 1 1/3 cups

One Serving Contains:
CALORIES 146.8; PROTEIN 0.3g; CARBOHYDRATE 10.4g; FAT 10.9g; SODIUM 5.6mg

BLACK BEAN HUMMUS

MANDI
2

Serves: 6 — Prep Time: 6 minutes

INGREDIENTS

1 15-ounce can black beans, no or low salt or 1 1/2 cups cooked beans, drained, (reserve liquid from canned beans or cooking liquid from cooked beans)

2 tablespoons fresh lemon juice

2 tablespoons *Dr. Fuhrman's VegiZest* or other no salt seasoning

2 tablespoons raw tahini

2 teaspoons Bragg Liquid Aminos or low sodium soy sauce

1/2 teaspoon ground cumin

1/2 clove garlic, chopped

pinch cayenne pepper, or to taste

pinch paprika, for garnish

DIRECTIONS

Blend all ingredients, except the paprika, in food processor with 2 table-spoons bean liquid. Process until smooth, scraping down the sides as needed. Add additional seasoning and liquid to taste.

Garnish with paprika.

Serve with raw vegetables like baby carrots, steamed asparagus spears, broccoli florets, zucchini, cucumber, and romaine lettuce leaves.

One Serving Contains:
CALORIES 88.2; PROTEIN 4.9g; CARBOHYDRATE 12.2g; FAT 2.6g; SODIUM 84.6mg

Blueberry Dressing/Dip

MANDI
7.5

Serves: 4 — Prep Time: 5 minutes

INGREDIENTS

2 cups frozen blueberries, thawed

1/4 cup unhulled sesame seeds

1/4 cup sunflower seeds

1/2 cup pomegranate juice

4 tablespoons *Dr. Fuhrman's Wild Blueberry Vinegar*

DIRECTIONS

Blend all ingredients in a high powered blender.

One Serving Contains:
CALORIES 164; PROTEIN 4.0g; CARBOHYDRATE 17.9g; FAT 9.4g; SODIUM 4.5mg

CAESAR SALAD DRESSING/DIP

Serves: 3 — Prep Time: 8 minutes

**MANDI
1.5**

INGREDIENTS

3 cloves garlic, roasted*

1/2 cup soy milk

1/4 cup raw cashew butter

1 tablespoon fresh lemon juice

1 tablespoon nutritional yeast (optional)

1 1/2 teaspoons Dijon mustard

dash black pepper

DIRECTIONS

Roast garlic. Remove skins and blend with the rest of the ingredients in a high powered blender until creamy and smooth.

To roast garlic; break the cloves apart. Leave the papery skins on. Roast at 350 degrees for about 25 minutes until mushy.

One Serving Contains:
CALORIES 154.3; PROTEIN 5.7g; CARBOHYDRATE 9.3g; FAT 11.3g; SODIUM 85.8mg

MAY BE USED FOR A VEGGIE DIP OR POUR OVER 2 CHOPPED HEADS (12 CUPS) OF ROMAINE LETTUCE FOR A CAESAR SALAD FOR TWO.

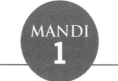

CASHEW-CURRANT DRESSING/DIP

Serves: 4 — Prep Time: 5 minutes

INGREDIENTS

1/4 cup raw cashews or 2 tablespoons raw cashew butter

1/3 cup soy milk

1/4 cup unsweetened applesauce

1/4 cup dried currants or raisins

DIRECTIONS

Blend the cashews or cashew butter with soy milk and applesauce in a high powered blender until smooth. Mix in currents or raisins.

One Serving Contains:
CALORIES 89.8; PROTEIN 2.8g; CARBOHYDRATE 12g; FAT 4.2g; SODIUM 13.1mg

CHOCOLATE DIP

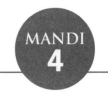

Serves: 8 — Prep Time: 15 minutes

INGREDIENTS

1 1/2 cups whole raw almonds or raw cashews

3/4 cup vanilla soy milk

2 cups organic baby spinach

2 cups frozen strawberries or blueberries

2/3 cup dates, pitted

3 tablespoons *Dr. Fuhrman's Cocoa Powder* or other natural cocoa powder

2 tablespoons Goji berries (optional)

1 teaspoon vanilla extract

1/2 raw beet or 2 tablespoons beet powder, to adjust color

DIRECTIONS

Blend nuts and soy milk until smooth. Add remaining ingredients and blend again.

May be eaten as a pudding or used as a dip for fresh fruit and vegetables.

One Serving Contains:
CALORIES 192.6; PROTEIN 7.8g; CARBOHYDRATE 11.9g; FAT 14.5g; SODIUM 31.1mg

CREAMY SESAME DRESSING/DIP

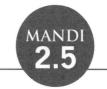

MANDI
2.5

Serves: 6 — Prep Time: 5 minutes

INGREDIENTS

2/3 cup unhulled sesame seeds, lightly toasted*

7 pitted dates

1/2 clove garlic

1 cup soy milk

2 tablespoons *Dr. Fuhrman's Riesling Raisin Vinegar*

1 tablespoon raw cashew butter

1 teaspoon sesame oil

DIRECTIONS

Blend all ingredients in high powered blender until smooth and creamy. Add additional soy milk to thin if necessary.

Lightly toast sesame seeds in a pan over medium heat for 3 minutes, shaking pan frequently.

One Serving Contains:
CALORIES 191.1; PROTEIN 6.1g; CARBOHYDRATE 16.1g; FAT 13.0g; SODIUM 24.9mg

DIJON DATE DRESSING/DIP

MANDI
2.5

Serves: 2 — Prep Time: 10 minutes

INGREDIENTS

1/2 cup water

3 tablespoons raw cashew butter

2 tablespoons *Dr. Fuhrman's Riesling Raisin Vinegar* or balsamic vinegar

1 tablespoon *Dr. Fuhrman's VegiZest* or other no salt seasoning

1 tablespoon Dijon mustard

8 deglet noor dates or 4 medjool dates

1-2 cloves garlic, minced

DIRECTIONS

Blend all dressing ingredients in a high powered blender.

One Serving Contains:
CALORIES 273.7; PROTEIN 6.1g; CARBOHYDRATE 37.6g; FAT 12g; SODIUM 209.3mg

DIJON PISTACHIO DRESSING /DIP

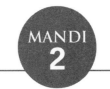

Serves: 2 — Prep Time: 5 minutes

INGREDIENTS

2/3 cup water

1/2 cup pistachio nuts, unsalted, preferably raw

2 tablespoons lemon juice

1 tablespoon ground flax seeds

2 teaspoons *Dr. Fuhrman's VegiZest*

1 teaspoon Dijon mustard

1/2 teaspoon Bragg Liquid Aminos or low sodium soy sauce

1/4 teaspoon garlic powder

2 deglet noor dates or 1 medjool date (optional)

DIRECTIONS

Blend all ingredients in a high powered blender until smooth and creamy.

One Serving Contains:
CALORIES 236.9; PROTEIN 8g; CARBOHYDRATE 21.3g; FAT 15.2g; SODIUM 137.6mg

EGGPLANT HUMMUS

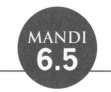

MANDI
6.5

Serves: 4 — Prep Time: 10 minutes

INGREDIENTS

1 medium eggplant, cut in half

1 cup cooked or canned garbanzo beans (chickpeas), low or no salt, drained

1/3 cup bean liquid (from the can of garbanzo beans) or water

4 tablespoons raw unhulled sesame seeds

2 tablespoons lemon juice

1 tablespoon dried chopped onions

4 cloves garlic, chopped fine

dash paprika and/or dried parsley for garnish (optional)

DIRECTIONS

Bake eggplant at 350 degrees for 45 minutes.

Let cool, remove skin & discard.

Blend all ingredients, including baked, peeled eggplant, in a high powered blender until creamy smooth.

One Serving Contains:
CALORIES 163.6; PROTEIN 7g; CARBOHYDRATE 24.1g; FAT 5.8g; SODIUM 8.1mg

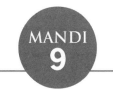

Garbanzo Guacamole

Serves: 2 — Prep Time: 20 minutes

INGREDIENTS

1/2 15-oz can garbanzo beans, no salt, drained

1 clove garlic, halved

1 tablespoon lemon juice

1 avocado, peeled and cubed

1 1/2 fresh green chili peppers, minced

1 cup chopped tomato

3/4 cup chopped green onions

1 teaspoon Bragg Liquid Aminos or low sodium soy sauce

assorted raw vegetables, cut up

DIRECTIONS

In food processor, puree beans and garlic with lemon juice.

Add avocado and chili peppers, pulsing until mixture is chunky.

Remove to bowl and stir in tomato, green onions, and liquid aminos.

Serve with raw vegetables.

One Serving Contains:
CALORIES 363.3; PROTEIN 15.8g; CARBOHYDRATE 47.2g; FAT 16.1g; SODIUM 147.9mg

GREEN VELVET DRESSING/DIP

MANDI
4

Serves: 4 — Prep Time: 10 minutes

INGREDIENTS

3/4 cup water

1/2 cup fresh lemon juice

1/2 cup raw tahini

1/4 cup chopped fresh parsley

1/4 cup chopped fresh dill

4 tablespoons raw cashews

2 tablespoons *Dr. Fuhrman's VegiZest*

1/2 tablespoon chopped fresh tarragon (optional)

2 teaspoons Bragg Liquid Aminos or low sodium soy sauce

2 cloves garlic, chopped

DIRECTIONS

Blend all ingredients in a high powered blender until smooth.

One Serving Contains:
CALORIES 241.3; PROTEIN 8.5g; CARBOHYDRATE 16g; FAT 18.2g; SODIUM 168.1mg

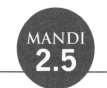

HOT PEPPER SALSA

Serves: 10 — Prep Time: 25 minutes

INGREDIENTS

3 large plum tomatoes, cut in fourths

1 medium onion, cut in fourths

4 cloves garlic, cut in half

1 14-ounce can whole or chopped tomatoes

1 jar roasted red peppers, low sodium, in vinegar (drained)

1/2 cup fresh cilantro

2 tablespoons red wine vinegar

1 long hot pepper

DIRECTIONS

Roast tomatoes, onions and garlic in a 400 degree oven for 10 minutes.

Remove from oven and place in a food processor. Add rest of ingredients and pulse to chop until desired consistency.

Yields: approx. 2 1/2 cups

One Serving Contains:
CALORIES 25.4; PROTEIN 2g; CARBOHYDRATE 5.8g; FAT 0.2g; SODIUM 62.1mg

ORANGE CASHEW DRESSING/DIP

Serves: 3 — Prep Time: 2 minutes

INGREDIENTS

2 oranges, peeled and quartered

1/3 cup raw cashews

2 tablespoons *Dr. Fuhrman's Blood Orange Vinegar*

1/2 teaspoon lemon juice (optional)

DIRECTIONS

Blend all ingredients in a high powered blender until smooth and creamy.

Add some orange juice to thin, if necessary.

One Serving Contains:
CALORIES 127.2; PROTEIN 3.0g; CARBOHYDRATE 14.9g; FAT 6.8g; SODIUM 2.6mg

ORANGE PEANUT DRESSING/DIP

MANDI
1.5

Serves: 4 — Prep Time: 5 minutes

INGREDIENTS

1/2 cup orange juice

1/4 cup rice vinegar

2 tablespoons peanut butter

1/8 cup raw cashew butter or almond butter

1 teaspoon Bragg Liquid Aminos or low sodium soy sauce

1/4 inch piece fresh ginger, peeled

1/4 clove garlic

DIRECTIONS

Blend all ingredients in a high powered blender until smooth.

One Serving Contains:
CALORIES 117.6; PROTEIN 3.8g; CARBOHYDRATE 7.8g; FAT 8.1g; SODIUM 99.7mg

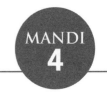

RED PEPPER SALSA

Serves: 4 — Prep Time: 10 minutes

INGREDIENTS

2 red bell peppers, stems removed

1/2 cup minced fennel

1 tablespoon red wine vinegar

1/2 tablespoon olive oil

1 1/2 teaspoons *Dr. Fuhrman's VegiZest*

1/2 teaspoon minced garlic

freshly ground black pepper, to taste

DIRECTIONS

Broil peppers on high until softened and brown on all sides, about 25 minutes, turning after 10 minutes. Enclose in a paper bag and let stand 10 minutes. Peel, seed, and chop peppers.

Mix fennel, vinegar, oil, VegiZest, garlic, and red peppers in medium bowl. Season with pepper.

Good served with endive leaves for dipping.

One Serving Contains:
CALORIES 37.5; PROTEIN 1g; CARBOHYDRATE 5g; FAT 1.9g; SODIUM 13.4mg

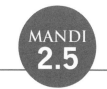

Russian Fig Dressing/Dip

Serves: 2 — Prep Time: 5 minutes

INGREDIENTS

4 tablespoons pasta sauce, no or low salt

3 tablespoons raw almond butter

2 tablespoons *Dr. Fuhrman's Black Fig Vinegar*

DIRECTIONS

Mash all ingredients together with a fork to blend.

One Serving Contains:
CALORIES 179.1; PROTEIN 3.9g; CARBOHYDRATE 10.8g; FAT 13.9g; SODIUM 8.9mg

SESAME FIG DRESSING

MANDI
2.5

Serves: 3 — Prep Time: 5 minutes

INGREDIENTS

1/4 cup water

1/4 cup raw tahini

2 tablespoons fig preserves

1 tablespoon sesame oil

1 tablespoon *Dr. Fuhrman's Black Fig Vinegar*

DIRECTIONS

Using a wire whisk or blender combine all ingredients together until smooth and creamy.

One Serving Contains:
CALORIES 183.5; PROTEIN 3.8g; CARBOHYDRATE 12.5g; FAT 14.2g; SODIUM 16.9mg

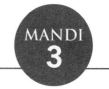

SPICY BEAN SPREAD/DIP

Serves: 4 — Prep Time: 10 minutes

INGREDIENTS

1 15-ounce can pinto beans, (no or low salt) reserving 1/2 of the liquid

1 teaspoon *Dr. Fuhrman's Black Fig Vinegar* or balsamic vinegar

1/2 teaspoon crushed red chili pepper

1/4 teaspoon garlic powder, or two garlic cloves, crushed

1 pinch turmeric

DIRECTIONS

In a blender or food processor, puree the beans with half the bean liquid and the vinegar.

Mix in the spices.

Serve with raw or lightly steamed vegetables or toasted pita bread with shredded raw greens.

One Serving Contains:
CALORIES 154.5; PROTEIN 9.6g; CARBOHYDRATE 28.3g; FAT 0.7g; SODIUM 1.4mg

STRAWBERRY DRESSING/SAUCE

MANDI
3.5

Serves: 3 — Prep Time: 5 minutes

INGREDIENTS

1/2 bag frozen strawberries, thawed or 1 pint fresh organic strawberries

1/2 cup vanilla soy milk

1 tablespoon date sugar, or 2 dates

DIRECTIONS

Blend all ingredients together in a high powered blender.

May be served over banana/fruit "ice cream", a fruit salad, or with a salad or steamed vegetables.

One Serving Contains:
CALORIES 62.9; PROTEIN 2.3g; CARBOHYDRATE 13g; FAT 0.9g; SODIUM 23.6mg

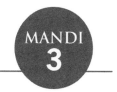

TAHINI DRESSING/DIP

Serves: 4 — Prep Time: 6 minutes

INGREDIENTS

1 cup water

1/2 cup raw tahini (pureed sesame seeds)

1/4 cup fresh lemon juice

1 tablespoon *Dr. Fuhrman's VegiZest*

1 teaspoon Bragg Liquid Aminos or low sodium soy sauce (optional)

6-8 pitted dates, to taste

1/2 medium banana

1 clove garlic, chopped

DIRECTIONS

Blend all ingredients together in a high powered blender
until smooth and creamy.

One Serving Contains:
CALORIES 229.9; PROTEIN 6.5g; CARBOHYDRATE 23.2g; FAT 14.5g; SODIUM 94.9mg

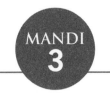

TASTY HUMMUS

Serves: 4 — Prep Time: 10 minutes

INGREDIENTS

1 cup cooked or canned garbanzo beans (low or no salt), reserving liquid

1/4 cup bean liquid or water

1/4 cup raw unhulled sesame seeds

1 tablespoon lemon juice

1 tablespoon *Dr. Fuhrman's VegiZest* or other no salt seasoning

1 teaspoon Bragg Liquid Aminos or low sodium soy sauce

1 teaspoon horseradish (optional)

1 small clove garlic, chopped

DIRECTIONS

Blend all ingredients in a high powered blender until creamy smooth.

This is a great spread or dip for raw and lightly steamed vegetables.

Yields: 1 cup

One Serving Contains:
CALORIES 127.2; PROTEIN 5.9g; CARBOHYDRATE 15.1g; FAT 5.5g; SODIUM 78.6mg

TOFU RANCH DRESSING/DIP

MANDI
1.5

Serves: 4 — Prep Time: 10 minutes

INGREDIENTS

6 ounces silken tofu

3 dates, pitted

1 clove garlic

1/4 cup finely chopped green onion

3 tablespoons water

2 tablespoons lemon juice

1 1/2 tablespoons Italian seasoning

1 tablespoon chopped fresh parsley

1 tablespoon chopped fresh dill

2 teaspoons Bragg Liquid Aminos or low sodium soy sauce

1 dash cayenne pepper (optional)

> USE AS A DRESSING, DIP, SPREAD OR MAYONNAISE SUBSTITUTE IN YOUR FAVORITE RECIPES.

DIRECTIONS

In a blender or food processor, combine all of the ingredients and process until smooth.

Transfer to an airtight container and store in the refrigerator for up to 5 days.

One Serving Contains:
CALORIES 62.6; PROTEIN 2.2g; CARBOHYDRATE 12.7g; FAT 1g; SODIUM 126.9mg

TOMATO ALMOND DRESSING/DIP

MANDI
3.5

Serves: 4 — Prep Time: 5 minutes

INGREDIENTS

1 cup pasta sauce, no or low salt

2 tablespoons almond butter

1 tablespoon balsamic vinegar

1 teaspoon *Dr. Fuhrman's Spicy Pecan Vinegar* (optional)

1/2 teaspoon crushed garlic or 1/4 teaspoon garlic powder

1/2 teaspoon onion powder or onion flakes

DIRECTIONS

Place pasta sauce and almond butter in a bowl and combine with a whisk.

Add vinegar, garlic, and onion powder.

Yields: approx 1 cup

One Serving Contains:
CALORIES 78.3; PROTEIN 2g; CARBOHYDRATE 7.4g; FAT 4.7g; SODIUM 8.5mg

Soups and Stews

Black Forest Cream of Mushroom Soup

MANDI
19

Serves: 8 — Prep Time: 30 minutes

INGREDIENTS

1/2 cup dried mixed mushrooms (optional)

2 pounds mixed fresh mushrooms (button, shiitake, cremini), sliced 1/4" thick

2 cloves garlic, minced or pressed

2 teaspoons herb de Provence

2 carrots, coarsely chopped

3 cups cauliflower florets, cut into small pieces

1 cup chopped organic celery

3 leeks, cut into ½ inch rounds

4 tablespoons *Dr. Fuhrman's VegiZest,* or other no salt seasoning

5 cups carrot juice

3 cups water

1/4 cup raw cashews

1 tablespoon lemon juice

1 tablespoon chopped fresh thyme

2 teaspoons chopped fresh rosemary

2 cans white beans, northern, navy, or cannellini (no salt)

1 5-oz bag organic baby spinach

1/4 cup chopped fresh parsley

continued...

BLACK FOREST
CREAM OF MUSHROOM SOUP *continued...*

DIRECTIONS

If using dried mushrooms, soak them in hot water to cover for 30 minutes and cut in pieces.

Heat 1/8 cup water in large sauté pan. Water sauté the fresh and dried mushrooms, garlic and dried herbs until tender and fragrant. Set aside.

In large soup pot, bring carrot juice, water, carrots, cauliflower, celery, leeks and VegiZest to a boil. Reduce heat and simmer until vegetables are tender, about 30 minutes.

Puree 1/2 vegetable soup in high powered blender; add cashews, lemon juice, and fresh herbs. Blend until smooth and creamy.

Add pureed soup back to soup pot along with mushrooms, beans, and spinach. Heat until spinach is wilted.

Serve garnished with fresh chopped parsley.

One Serving Contains:
CALORIES 305.9; PROTEIN 18.7g; CARBOHYDRATE 57.1g; FAT 3.1g; SODIUM 131.7mg

CHUNKY SWEET POTATO STEW

Serves: 2 — Prep Time: 25 minutes

INGREDIENTS

1 tablespoon olive oil

1 onion, thickly sliced

2 large garlic cloves, chopped

1 14-ounce can stewed tomatoes with juice (low or no salt)

1 large sweet potato, peeled, cut into 1/2 inch pieces

1/2 cup canned garbanzo beans (chick peas)
  or white kidney beans (low or no salt), drained

3/4 teaspoon dried rosemary

1 medium zucchini, cut into 1/2 inch thick rounds,
  or cut into bite-sized pieces

black pepper, to taste

Mrs. Dash seasoning, to taste

DIRECTIONS

Heat olive oil in large saucepan over medium heat. Add onion and cook about 5 minutes, until slightly softened, separating slices into rings. Add garlic and cook 1 minute.

Mix in stewed tomatoes with juice, sweet potatoes, garbanzo beans and rosemary. Bring mixture to a simmer, stirring occasionally. Cover and cook 5 minutes. Add zucchini. Cover and cook until sweet potatoes are tender, about 15 minutes, stirring occasionally.

Season to taste with pepper and/or Mrs. Dash.

One Serving Contains:
CALORIES 286.5; PROTEIN 9g; CARBOHYDRATE 48g; FAT 8.5g; SODIUM 73.1mg

DR. FUHRMAN'S FAMOUS
ANTI-CANCER SOUP

MANDI
29.5

Serves: 10 — Prep Time: 20 minutes

INGREDIENTS

1 cup dried split peas and/or beans

4 cups water

4 medium onions

6-10 medium zucchini

3 leek stalks

2 bunches kale, collards or other greens, chopped,
   tough stems and center ribs cut off and discarded

5 pounds carrots (4-5 cups juice)*

2 bunches organic celery (2 cups juice)*

2 tablespoons *Dr. Fuhrman's VegiZest*

1 tablespoon Mrs. Dash

1 cup raw cashews

8 ounces mushrooms (shiitake, cremini and/or oyster) chopped

DIRECTIONS

Place the beans and water in a very large pot over low heat.

Add whole onions, whole zucchini and whole leeks to the pot along with
chopped kale. Add carrot juice, celery juice and VegiZest (or Mrs Dash).

Simmer mixture until onions, zucchini and leeks are soft, about 20
minutes. Remove the soft onions, zucchini, and leeks from the pot along
with some of the soup liquid, being careful to leave the beans and some
of the kale in the pot.

continued...

Dr. Fuhrman's Famous
Anti-Cancer Soup *continued...*

Using a blender or food processor, completely blend/puree the onions, zucchini, and leeks. Add more soup liquid and the cashews to the mixture, and blend in. Return the blended, creamy mixture back to the pot. Add the mushrooms and simmer another 30 minutes or until beans are soft.

Juice carrots and celery in a juice extractor. Fresh juiced organic carrots are necessary to maximize the flavor of this soup.

One Serving Contains:
CALORIES 304.1; PROTEIN 14.4g; CARBOHYDRATE 52.4g; FAT 7g; SODIUM 134.6mg

FAST BLACK BEAN SOUP

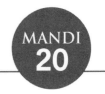

MANDI
20

Serves: 5 — Prep Time: 15 minutes

INGREDIENTS

2 15-ounce cans black beans, no or low salt

2 cups frozen mixed vegetables

2 cups frozen corn

2 cups frozen chopped broccoli florets

2 cups carrot juice*

1 cup water

1 15-ounce can prepared black bean soup, no or low salt**

1/4 cup chopped cilantro (optional)

1/8 teaspoon chili powder, or to taste

1 cup chopped fresh tomatoes

1 avocado, chopped or mashed (optional)

1/2 cup chopped green onions (optional)

1/4 cup raw pumpkin seeds, lightly toasted (optional)

DIRECTIONS

Combine black beans, mixed vegetables, corn, broccoli, carrot juice, water, soup, cilantro, and chili powder in a soup pot. Bring to a boil and simmer on low for 30 minutes. Stir in fresh tomatoes and heat through.

Serve topped with avocado, green onions, and pumpkin seeds, if desired.

*Carrot juice may be made in a juice extractor. Fresh or bottled carrot juice is also sold in many health food stores.

** See Purchasing Guidelines on page 90.

One Serving Contains:
CALORIES 402.7; PROTEIN 25.1g; CARBOHYDRATE 79.9g; FAT 2.2g; SODIUM 135.0mg

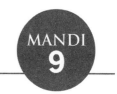

FRENCH MINTED PEA SOUP

Serves: 3 — Prep Time: 20 minutes

INGREDIENTS

10 ounces green peas, frozen

1 small onion, chopped

1 clove garlic, chopped

1 bunch fresh mint leaves (save a few leaves for garnish)
or 10 dried leaves

3 tablespoons *Dr. Fuhrman's VegiZest*,
or other no salt soup base seasoning

3 cups water

3 dates, pitted

1/2 cup raw cashews

1/2 tablespoon Spike (no salt seasoning), or to taste

4 teaspoons lemon juice

4 cups shredded romaine lettuce or chopped organic baby spinach

2 tablespoons fresh snipped chives (optional)

DIRECTIONS

Simmer peas, onions, garlic, mint and VegiZest in water for about 7 minutes.

Pour pea mixture into a high powered blender. Add remaining ingredients except for the lettuce and chives. Blend until smooth and creamy.

Add lettuce or spinach and let it wilt in hot liquid.

Pour into bowls and garnish with chives and mint leaves.

One Serving Contains:
CALORIES 287.8; PROTEIN 13g; CARBOHYDRATE 41.5g; FAT 10.2g; SODIUM 170.8mg

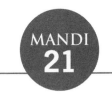

GAZPACHO SUMMER SOUP

Serves: 3   —   Prep Time: 20 minutes

INGREDIENTS

1 large cucumber, peeled and sliced into large pieces

1 large red bell pepper, seeded and sliced into large pieces

1 14-ounce diced or chopped tomatoes, no salt added

1 cup roasted red peppers, in vinegar, low sodium (drained)

2 cups tomato juice, low sodium

1 12-ounce jar mild or medium salsa, low sodium

1/2 cup fresh cilantro

2 tablespoons red wine vinegar

1 tablespoon *Dr. Fuhrman's VegiZest*

cucumber slices (optional)

DIRECTIONS

Place cucumbers and fresh red bell peppers in a food processor. Pulse until chopped in small pieces. Add canned tomatoes and roasted red peppers. Pulse a couple of more times until finely chopped. Add tomato juice and rest of ingredients and pulse until well mixed.

Cover and chill for at least 2 hours for flavors to mingle.

Before serving, garnish with cucumber slices, if desired. Serve chilled.

One Serving Contains:
CALORIES 136.2; PROTEIN 9.4g; CARBOHYDRATE 29.1g; FAT 1.1g; SODIUM 826.1mg

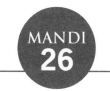

HEARTY GINGER LENTIL SOUP

Serves: 7 — Prep Time: 35 minutes

INGREDIENTS

8 cups carrot juice*

4 cups water

1 cup dried lentils (do not soak)

1/2 cup uncooked brown rice

2 zucchini, finely chopped

2 carrots, chopped

1 red bell pepper, finely chopped

1 onion, finely chopped

6 cloves garlic, minced or pressed

3 tablespoons grated fresh ginger root

3 tablespoons *Dr. Fuhrman's VegiZest*

1 teaspoon ground coriander

1/2 teaspoon ground cumin

1/8 teaspoon ground allspice

2 sweet potatoes, peeled and cut into 1" cubes

2 bunches Swiss chard leaves and stems, chopped

1/2 cup chopped fresh parsley

continued...

HEARTY GINGER LENTIL SOUP   *continued...*

DIRECTIONS

Place all ingredients, except for the sweet potatoes, swiss chard and parsley, in a soup pot. Bring to a boil, cover and simmer for 40 minutes. Add the potatoes and simmer for 15 minutes. Add the chard and simmer for 10 minutes. Serve topped with chopped parsley.

*Carrot juice may be made in a juice extractor. Fresh or bottled carrot juice is also sold in many health food stores.

One Serving Contains:
CALORIES 346; PROTEIN 14.6g; CARBOHYDRATE 72.4g; FAT 1.5g; SODIUM 234mg

Hearty Vegetable Stew

MANDI
36

Serves: 8 — Prep Time: 30 minutes

INGREDIENTS

> 1/2 cup dried lentils, rinsed
>
> 1/2 cup split peas, rinsed
>
> 4 cups water
>
> 1/2 head broccoli florets, bite-sized
>
> 1/2 head cauliflower florets, bite-sized
>
> 3 medium red bell peppers, coarsely chopped
>
> 1 medium beet, peeled and cubed
>
> 1 small eggplant, peeled if desired and cubed
>
> 1 cup carrots, cut 1/2 inch thick
>
> 1 cup organic celery, coarsely chopped
>
> 1 large onion or 3 leeks, chopped or sliced
>
> 5 cloves garlic, chopped
>
> 2 bunches kale, washed, leaves removed from stems and chopped
>
> 1 24-ounce can tomatoes, chopped or crushed, low or no sodium
>
> 8 tablespoons *Dr. Fuhrman's VegiZest* or other no salt seasoning
>
> 2 medium zucchini, cubed
>
> 2 cups carrot juice
>
> 4 teaspoons cinnamon (optional)
>
> 1/2 cup raw cashews

continued...

HEARTY VEGETABLE STEW *continued...*

DIRECTIONS

Place lentils, split peas and water in a large soup pot and begin to simmer.

Prepare vegetables and add all ingredients, except for zucchini, carrot juice, cinnamon and cashews, to simmering lentils and peas. If necessary, add more water to keep from scorching. Simmer covered for 30 minutes or until vegetables, lentils, and peas are tender.

Add zucchini, carrot juice, and cinnamon and simmer for another 30 minutes.

To make a creamy, chunky stew, blend 1/4 of cooked vegetable mixture with cashews in a high powered blender until smooth. Add blended mixture back into stew.

One Serving Contains:
CALORIES 314; PROTEIN 19.7g; CARBOHYDRATE 57.6g; FAT 5.2g; SODIUM 165.1mg

HIGH CRUCIFEROUS VEGETABLE STEW

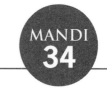

Serves: 10 — Prep Time: 45 minutes

INGREDIENTS

4 cups water

20 ounces carrot juice

1/2 cup dried split peas

1/2 cup dried lentils (red lentils make a prettier soup)

1/2 cup aduki (adzuki) beans, soaked overnight
  or use canned (no or low salt)

1 bunch kale, stems removed and discarded
  and leaves coarsely chopped

1 bunch collard greens, fresh or frozen, coarsely chopped

1 bunch broccoli, cut into florets

1/2 pound Brussels sprouts, fresh or frozen (if large cut in half)

1/2 pound shiitake mushrooms, sliced in half

10 ounces organic celery stalks, sliced in 1-inch pieces

3 leeks, coarsely chopped

3 carrots, sliced in 1-inch pieces

3 parsnips, sliced in 1-inch pieces

3 onions, chopped

4 medium zucchini, cubed

4 cloves garlic, chopped or 2 tsp garlic powder

1 28-ounce can tomatoes, low or no salt

continued...

HIGH CRUCIFEROUS VEGETABLE STEW   *continued...*

4 tablespoons *Dr. Fuhrman's VegiZest* or other no salt seasoning

2 tablespoons Mrs. Dash seasoning

1/2 bunch fresh parsley leaves, chopped

1 cup broccoli sprouts (optional)

DIRECTIONS

In large soup pot place all ingredients, except parsley and sprouts. Cover and bring to a simmer. Simmer until adzuki beans are tender. If using canned adzuki beans simmer until vegetables are tender and flavors blend, about 1 hour.

In a food processor or high powered blender, blend 1/4 of soup until smooth. Add back to soup pot and stir in parsley and broccoli sprouts.

One Serving Contains:
CALORIES 289.6; PROTEIN 15.4g; CARBOHYDRATE 59.9g; FAT 1.6g; SODIUM 134.1mg

QUICK AND CREAMY VEGETABLE BEAN SOUP

Serves: 8 — Prep Time: 15 minutes

INGREDIENTS

4 cups prepared tomato soup, natural or organic, no or low sodium*

2 cups frozen broccoli florets

2 cups frozen chopped organic spinach

2 cups carrot juice

1 cup frozen chopped onions

4 cans cannellini beans or other white beans, no salt

3 fresh tomatoes, chopped

1 bunch fresh basil, chopped

4 tablespoons *Dr. Fuhrman's VegiZest*

1 teaspoon garlic powder

Italian seasoning, to taste

1/2 cup raw cashew nuts

1/4 cup pine nuts

DIRECTIONS

In soup pot, combine all ingredients, except cashews and pine nuts. Cover and simmer for 30-40 minutes.

In high powered blender, blend 1/4 of soup mixture with cashew nuts. Add back to soup pot.

Serve with pine nuts sprinkled on top.

*See Purchasing Guidelines on page 90.

One Serving Contains:
CALORIES 355.3; PROTEIN 19.5g; CARBOHYDRATE 57.3g; FAT 8.7g; SODIUM 111.3mg

SPEEDY VEGETABLES AND BEANS SOUP

Serves: 10 — Prep Time: 15 minutes

INGREDIENTS

1 pound frozen Asian vegetables

1 pound frozen broccoli florets

1 pound frozen mixed vegetables

1 pound frozen collard greens

2 cups frozen corn

1 cup frozen onions

7 cups carrot juice

3 cups water

1 1/2 cups sun-dried tomatoes, snipped in half

1 cup adzuki beans, low or no salt, including some bean liquid

1 cup red beans, low or no salt, including some bean liquid

2 15-ounce cans lentils, low or no salt

4 cloves garlic, chopped

4 tablespoons *Dr. Fuhrman's VegiZest* or other no salt seasoning

1 tablespoon Spike, no salt

2 teaspoons chili powder

8 ounces organic baby spinach or coarsely chopped organic spinach

DIRECTIONS

In a large soup pot combine all ingredients, except the fresh spinach. Cover and simmer for 1 hour, stirring occasionally. Add more water if a thinner soup is desired.

Turn off heat and stir in spinach to wilt.

One Serving Contains:
CALORIES 370.8; PROTEIN 21.8g; CARBOHYDRATE 74.6g; FAT 2.1g; SODIUM 340.3mg

TOMATO BEAN BARLEY SOUP

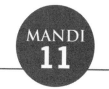

Serves: 6 — Prep Time: 30 minutes

INGREDIENTS

7 cups vegetable broth (low sodium)

1 cup water

1 cup dried barley

1 teaspoon olive oil

1 tablespoon water

1 cup chopped onions

1/2 cup chopped organic celery

3 medium carrots, chopped

6 cloves garlic, chopped

1 14 1/2-ounce can chopped tomatoes (no or low salt)

1 15-ounce can kidney beans (no or low sodium), drained

1/4 teaspoon crushed red pepper flakes

8 packed cups organic baby spinach

1/4 teaspoon black pepper

DIRECTIONS

In a large soup pot, bring vegetable broth, water, and barley to a boil. Reduce heat, cover and simmer for 20 minutes or until barley is tender.

Meanwhile, heat oil and 1 tablespoon water in a pan. Add onions, celery, carrots, garlic, tomatoes, beans, and red pepper flakes. Cover and simmer over low heat for 15 minutes or until vegetables are tender.

Add vegetable/bean mixture to barley pot, stir in spinach and pepper and simmer an additional 5 minutes or until spinach is wilted.

One Serving Contains:
CALORIES 329; PROTEIN 14.4g; CARBOHYDRATE 67.1g; FAT 2.8g; SODIUM 228.4mg

WEST AFRICAN LENTIL OKRA STEW

MANDI
30.5

Serves: 8 — Prep Time: 20 minutes

INGREDIENTS

2 cups red lentils

2 tablespoons tomato paste

1/2 cup smooth natural no-salt peanut butter at room temperature

4 tablespoons *Dr. Fuhrman's VegiZest*

4 cups carrot juice

2 cups frozen chopped onion

16 ounces frozen okra, thawed and cut in half crosswise

16 ounces frozen chopped kale or collard greens

1 15-ounce can whole no-salt crushed or chopped tomatoes

1 medium sweet potato, chopped

4 cloves garlic, minced or pressed

3 teaspoons chili powder

pinch cayenne pepper

DIRECTIONS

In large saucepan, simmer red lentils in 3 cups of water for 15 minutes.

In mixing bowl, whisk tomato paste, peanut butter, VegiZest and carrot juice, then add to simmering lentils. Add remaining ingredients and bring to a boil. Reduce heat, cover and simmer for about 20 minutes.

Uncover and simmer another 20 minutes.

One Serving Contains:
CALORIES 413.6; PROTEIN 23g; CARBOHYDRATE 65.2g; FAT 9.5g; SODIUM 137.9mg

Non-Vegan Dishes

Creole Chicken with Spinach and Rice

MANDI
13.5

Serves: 4 — Prep Time: 20 minutes

INGREDIENTS

1 cup brown rice, uncooked

1/4 teaspoon chili powder

olive oil (small amount)

2 skinless, boneless chicken breast halves, thin sliced crosswise

1 1/2 cups chopped organic celery

1 cup chopped canned tomatoes, (no salt)

10 ounces frozen spinach

1 cup chili sauce (low salt)

1/4 cup chopped onion

1 large green pepper, chopped

2 cloves garlic, minced

1 tablespoon chopped fresh basil or 1 teaspoon dried

1 tablespoon chopped fresh parsley or 1 teaspoon dried

1/4 teaspoon dried crushed red pepper

continued...

CREOLE CHICKEN
WITH SPINACH AND RICE   *continued...*

DIRECTIONS

Cook brown rice according to package directions, adding chili powder to cooking water.

Using a paper towel moistened with olive oil, lightly coat a deep nonstick skillet and heat. Cook thin strips of chicken on medium high, turning occasionally, for 3-5 minutes until no longer pink.

Add remaining ingredients, bring to a boil and reduce heat to medium. Simmer covered for 10 minutes.

Serve over seasoned brown rice.

One Serving Contains:
CALORIES 359; PROTEIN 22.9g; CARBOHYDRATE 65.3g; FAT 3g; SODIUM 148.1mg

DIJON CHICKEN

MANDI
2.5

Serves: 2 — Prep Time: 10 minutes

INGREDIENTS

2 boneless and skinless chicken breasts

4 tablespoons fresh lime juice

2 tablespoons vegan Worcestershire sauce (found in health food stores)

4 teaspoons Dijon mustard

2 cloves garlic, minced

DIRECTIONS

Trim all fat from chicken breasts.

Mix together lime juice, Worcestershire sauce, Dijon mustard, and garlic.

Reserve half and pour the rest over chicken and marinate for 1/2 hour.

Broil on low or grill for 7 minutes per side or until cooked through. Serve with rest of marinade spooned over top.

Pair this recipe with California Creamed Kale or Lemon Zest Spinach.

One Serving Contains:
CALORIES 163.3; PROTEIN 27.6g; CARBOHYDRATE 6.9g; FAT 1.5g; SODIUM 484.4mg

EGG AND VEGETABLE SCRAMBLE

MANDI
21

Serves: 1 — Prep Time: 15 minutes

INGREDIENTS

2 eggs

2 tablespoons unsweetened soy milk

1/2 medium bell pepper, diced

2 green onions, chopped

1/2 cup diced fresh tomatoes

1/2 cup diced fresh mushrooms

1 tablespoon *Dr. Fuhrman's VegiZest* or other no salt seasoning

1 teaspoon Spike or other no salt seasoning

4 ounces organic spinach, coarsely chopped or baby spinach

DIRECTIONS

Beat eggs with soy milk.

Water sauté* the peppers, onions, tomatoes, mushrooms, VegiZest, and Spike until vegetables are tender. Add spinach to wilt.

Cook most water out of vegetables, then add eggs and scramble until cooked through.

To water sauté: heat 1/8 cup water in sauté pan and add vegetables. Cook until tender, adding more water if needed.

One Serving Contains:
CALORIES 252.9; PROTEIN 24.7g; CARBOHYDRATE 20.4g; FAT 11.5g; SODIUM 299.6mg

FILET OF SOLE WITH MANGO SALSA

MANDI
3.5

Serves: 4 — Prep Time: 15 minutes

INGREDIENTS

1 ripe mango, peeled, cut into small pieces

3 green onions, chopped

2 tablespoons chopped fresh cilantro

1 tablespoon fresh lemon juice

2 teaspoons chopped, seeded fresh jalapeno chili

4 pieces filet of sole (or flounder)

DIRECTIONS

To prepare salsa, combine first five ingredients in bowl. Let stand at room temperature 10 minutes to 2 hours.

Preheat broiler. Lightly coat a broiler pan using a paper towel moistened with olive oil. Broil fish 4 inches from heat source until just cooked through, about five minutes or until fish flakes easily with a fork.

Spoon salsa over fish.

One Serving Contains:
CALORIES 142.5; PROTEIN 21.9g; CARBOHYDRATE 10.2g; FAT 1.5g; SODIUM 96mg

GARDEN EGGS AND TOFU WITH SALSA

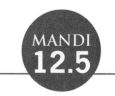

MANDI
12.5

Serves: 3 — Prep Time: 25 minutes

INGREDIENTS

1/2 medium onion, diced

1 medium zucchini, grated

1 carrot, grated

2 cups chopped Swiss chard or organic spinach

1/2 medium tomato, diced

2 cloves garlic, pressed

2 teaspoons herb de Provence (dried French herbs)

1 cup firm tofu

1/8 teaspoon curry powder, or more to taste

6 large eggs, beaten

1/4 cup prepared salsa, low sodium

1 ounce mozzarella cheese substitute, grated

6 sprouted grain tortillas (optional)

continued...

GARDEN EGGS AND TOFU
WITH SALSA   *continued...*

DIRECTIONS

In a large sauté pan, water sauté* the onion, zucchini, carrot, and Swiss chard for about 2 minutes. Add the tomato, garlic, and herbs. Cook, stirring for about 2 minutes, until the vegetables begin to soften.

Squeeze water out of tofu and crumble.

Scatter the tofu over the vegetables and sprinkle with curry powder. Mix with vegetables and cook over high heat until water is cooked away.

Reduce the heat to low and stir in the eggs, mixing well so the vegetables and tofu bind with the eggs. Continue stirring, until the eggs are cooked.

Top with salsa and grated cheese.

*To water sauté: heat 1/8 cup water in sauté pan and add vegetables. Cook until tender, adding more water if needed.

One Serving Contains:
CALORIES 332.8; PROTEIN 30.1g; CARBOHYDRATE 17.1g; FAT 18.4g; SODIUM 361mg

PASTA WITH SHRIMP AND ARTICHOKES

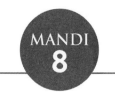

MANDI
8

Serves: 4 — Prep Time: 30 minutes

INGREDIENTS

1 tablespoon olive oil

1 medium onion, chopped

3 garlic cloves, minced

1/4 cup chopped fresh basil or 4 teaspoons dried

2 tablespoons chopped fresh oregano or 2 teaspoons dried

1/4 teaspoon dried crushed red pepper

2 teaspoons garlic powder

1 14-ounce can diced tomatoes, no salt

2 large tomatoes, seeded and diced

1 9-ounce package frozen artichoke hearts, thawed

1 tablespoon fresh lemon juice

3/4 pound whole wheat spaghetti

1 pound uncooked medium shrimp, peeled and deveined

continued...

PASTA WITH SHRIMP AND ARTICHOKES   *continued...*

DIRECTIONS

Heat oil in heavy large skillet over medium heat. Add onion and garlic; sauté until tender, about 5 minutes. Add basil, oregano, dried red pepper, and garlic powder and stir 1 minute.

Add canned and fresh diced tomatoes, artichoke hearts and lemon juice and simmer until sauce thickens slightly and artichokes are tender, about 30 minutes.

Cook spaghetti in large pot of boiling water until tender but still firm to bite. Drain, reserving 1 cup of cooking water.

Meanwhile, bring sauce to a simmer. Stir in shrimp and simmer until just cooked through, about 5 minutes.

Add spaghetti to sauce and toss to coat. Add reserved cooking liquid as necessary if pasta is too dry.

One Serving Contains:
CALORIES 522.1; PROTEIN 43.3g; CARBOHYDRATE 81.4g; FAT 7.3g; SODIUM 214.8mg

THIS RECIPE CAN ALSO BE MADE USING 1/2 WHOLE WHEAT PASTA AND 1/2 SPAGHETTI SQUASH.

Salsa Salmon Over Wilted Greens

Serves: 4   —   Prep Time: 30 minutes

INGREDIENTS

1 1/4 pounds salmon (wild or Icelandic farm-raised),
  cut into 4-oz. portions and skin removed

2 lemons, juiced

4 cloves garlic, pressed

3 teaspoons Spike no salt seasoning

water

3 medium zucchini, chopped

3 cloves garlic, pressed

6 Roma tomatoes, cut into 1/2" cubes

2 teaspoons *Dr. Fuhrman's VegiZest,*
  or other no salt seasoning

3 tablespoons chopped fresh basil

16 ounces fresh organic spinach or mixed field greens

continued...

SALSA SALMON
OVER WILTED GREENS   *continued...*

DIRECTIONS

Combine salmon with lemon juice, garlic and spike and marinate for 10 minutes.

To prepare Vegetable Salsa, heat 1/8 cup water in a large skillet, add zucchini and garlic and sauté for 5 minutes, adding more water if necessary until zucchini is tender. Add the tomatoes and VegiZest and simmer uncovered over medium high heat, stirring occasionally, until very little liquid remains. Toss in 2 tablespoons of basil. Place mixture in bowl and set aside.

In same skillet, barely wilt greens in small amount of water.
Remove from heat.

SALMON MAY BE DONE UNDER A BROILER ON HIGH HEAT, ABOUT 4 MINUTES ON EACH SIDE, IF DESIRED.

Salmon: Heat grill on high with lid closed for 10 minutes until very hot. Grill fish with lid closed on high for about 5 minutes or until nicely browned. Turn fish and remove skin if it was not previously removed.

Grill uncovered on medium high for at least another 3-7 minutes (depending upon thickness) or until cooked through.

Serve on bed of wilted greens and top with the vegetable salsa and the remaining basil.

One Serving Contains:
CALORIES 329; PROTEIN 40.5g; CARBOHYDRATE 19.1g; FAT 13.1g; SODIUM 117.9mg

SCRAMBLED EGGS
WITH SPINACH & TOMATOES

MANDI
6.5

Serves: 1 — Prep Time: 5 minutes

INGREDIENTS

2 eggs

2 tablespoons soy milk

1 1/2 teaspoons Spike no salt seasoning

olive oil (small amount)

1 cup organic baby spinach

1/4 cup halved cherry tomato

DIRECTIONS

Using a fork or wire whisk, scramble eggs, soy milk, and seasoning together.

Using a paper towel moistened with olive oil, lightly coat skillet. Pour egg mixture into warm skillet and add spinach and cherry tomatoes. Mix together over medium heat until eggs are done and spinach is wilted.

One Serving Contains:
CALORIES 183.9; PROTEIN 15.7g; CARBOHYDRATE 7.3g; FAT 10.8g; SODIUM 185.3mg

SOUTHWESTERN CHICKEN

Serves: 4 — Prep Time: 15 minutes

INGREDIENTS

1 cup salsa, low sodium

1 cup black beans or red kidney beans, low or no sodium

1 cup fresh or frozen sweet corn

2 tablespoons fresh chopped cilantro

2 skinless, boneless chicken breasts

DIRECTIONS

Preheat oven to 350 degrees.

Mix salsa, beans, corn, and cilantro together.

Spoon 1/2 of the salsa mixture over the chicken and marinade for at least one hour.

Bake chicken for 30 minutes or until cooked through.

Slice the chicken breasts and top with remaining salsa mixture.

One Serving Contains:
CALORIES 240.7; PROTEIN 33.3g; CARBOHYDRATE 22.9g; FAT 2.1g; SODIUM 468.2mg

SPICED HADDOCK OR TILAPIA

MANDI
2

Serves: 4 — Prep Time: 20 minutes

INGREDIENTS

1 tablespoon olive oil

1/4 cup onion, minced

2 cloves garlic, minced

1 1/2 teaspoons paprika

4 4-ounce haddock or tilapia fillets

2 tablespoons fresh dill, chopped

6 cloves garlic

1 tablespoon fresh lemon juice

DIRECTIONS

Add oil to a nonstick cooking pan. Place over medium-high heat until hot. Add onion and garlic; cook, stirring constantly, until soft.

Stir in paprika. Remove from heat and let cool.

Spread onion mixture on both sides of fillets. Sprinkle with dill.

Lightly coat a broiler pan using a paper towel moistened with olive oil. Broil fillets and garlic cloves on high 3 inches from heat for 8 minutes or until fish flakes easily when tested with a fork.

Sprinkle with lemon juice and garnish with broiled garlic cloves.

Braised Bok Choy makes a quick and delicious side dish.

One Serving Contains:
CALORIES 144.8; PROTEIN 22.1g; CARBOHYDRATE 3.7g; FAT 4.3g; SODIUM 79.1mg

STEAK AND ROASTED VEGETABLE SALAD

MANDI 14.5

Serves: 4 — Prep Time: 35 minutes

INGREDIENTS

olive oil (small amount)

1 medium zucchini, cut diagonally into 1 inch pieces

1 medium fennel, cut into 1 inch wedges

1 large red pepper, cut into 1 inch strips

1 medium red onion, cut into 1 inch wedges

16 medium shiitake mushrooms, stems removed

2 tablespoons balsamic vinegar

2 large cloves garlic, minced

1 teaspoon dried crushed rosemary

1/8 teaspoon black pepper

3/4 pound beef tenderloin steaks, flank steak or boneless chicken breasts,

12 cups mixed salad greens

> FOR A VEGETARIAN DISH, THE MEAT MAY BE LEFT OUT OR YOU MAY USE STRIPS OF TOFU THAT HAVE BEEN BAKED.

BALSAMIC VINAIGRETTE

1/4 cup water

4 tablespoons olive oil

3 tablespoons roasted garlic rice vinegar

2 tablespoons balsamic vinegar

2 tablespoons 100% grape fruit spread or raisins

2 cloves garlic, pressed

continued...

STEAK AND ROASTED VEGETABLE SALAD   *continued...*

1/2 teaspoon dried oregano

1/4 teaspoon dried basil

1/4 teaspoon onion powder

DIRECTIONS

Preheat oven to 400 degrees.

Lightly coat a large baking pan with olive oil using a paper towel moistened with olive oil. Place vegetables in pan.

In a small bowl combine vinegar, minced garlic, rosemary, and black pepper and toss with vegetables. Roast in oven for 18-20 minutes until tender, stirring once.

Blend all vinaigrette ingredients together in a blender, or, if using the fruit spread, you can use a wire whisk to mix thoroughly.

Heat a large nonstick skillet over medium heat until hot.

Trim fat from meat and place in skillet. Cook 12-15 minutes depending on desired degree of doneness, turning once. (Meat may also be grilled, if desired)

Slice meat into thin strips.

Arrange meat and roasted vegetables over salad greens.

Serve immediately with dressing drizzled on top.

One Serving Contains:
CALORIES 452.3; PROTEIN 30.1g; CARBOHYDRATE 38g; FAT 21.3g; SODIUM 115.9mg

TURKEY SPINACH BURGERS

MANDI
8

Serves: 5 — Prep Time: 15 minutes

INGREDIENTS

1 pound ground turkey breast

10 ounces frozen, chopped spinach, defrosted and drained

1/4 cup dried bread crumbs

1/4 cup chopped onion

2 tablespoons chopped fresh parsley

1 1/2 tablespoons vegan Worcestershire sauce (found in health food stores)

1 teaspoon hot sauce

DIRECTIONS

Combine the ground turkey, spinach, bread crumbs, onions, parsley, Worcestershire sauce, and hot sauce in a large bowl. Mix well.

Divide turkey mixture into 5 equal portions and form into patties.

Coat grill rack or broiler pan with cooking spray.

Grill or broil until nicely browned on both sides and cooked through, about 7 minutes per side.

One Serving Contains:
CALORIES 181.3; PROTEIN 18.9g; CARBOHYDRATE 8.2g; FAT 8.2g; SODIUM 242.7mg

TURKEY-VEGETABLE MEATLOAF

MANDI
8.5

Serves: 8 — Prep Time: 20 minutes

INGREDIENTS

2 pounds ground turkey

1 cup quick oats (not instant)

10 ounces frozen organic chopped spinach, thawed and drained

1 large carrot, grated

1 medium green pepper, chopped

1 medium onion, chopped

2 eggs

2 large cloves garlic, minced

6 tablespoons ketchup, low sodium

2 tablespoons vegan Worcestershire sauce (found in health food stores)

1 tablespoon chopped fresh basil

1 teaspoon Dijon mustard

1 teaspoon Italian herb seasoning

1/2 teaspoon marjoram

1/4 teaspoon black pepper

1 14-ounce can chopped tomatoes, no salt added, drained

1 tablespoon ketchup (low sodium)

continued...

Turkey-Vegetable Meatloaf   *continued...*

DIRECTIONS

Preheat oven to 350 degrees.

Mix ground turkey and oats together. Add remaining ingredients except for half of the tomatoes and ketchup. Mix well to combine.

Shape into loaf and place in a large loaf pan or spread in a tube pan.

Top with remaining tomatoes mixed with 1 tablespoon of ketchup.

Bake for 1 hour 15 minutes until meat is cooked through.

One Serving Contains:

CALORIES 320; PROTEIN 28.6g; CARBOHYDRATE 25.8g; FAT 12.4g; SODIUM 229.8mg

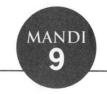

VEGETABLE OMELET

Serves: 2 — Prep Time: 10 minutes

INGREDIENTS

olive oil (small amount)

1 medium onion, diced

1 medium green or red peppers, diced

1 cup fresh shiitake mushrooms, stems removed and chopped

1 cup diced tomatoes

1/4 teaspoon dried basil

4 eggs, beaten

black pepper, to taste

DIRECTIONS

Using a paper towel moistened with olive oil, lightly coat skillet. Sauté the onions, peppers, mushrooms and tomatoes over medium heat for 10 minutes until tender.

Add basil and eggs and cook over med/high heat until done, about 8 minutes, turning over with spatula occasionally.

Sprinkle with black pepper.

One Serving Contains:
CALORIES 239; PROTEIN 19g; CARBOHYDRATE 22.1g; FAT 10.6g; SODIUM 162.6mg

VEGAN DISHES

ARTICHOKES WITH DIPPING SAUCE

MANDI 2.5

Serves: 6 — Prep Time: 15 minutes

INGREDIENTS

6 large artichokes

2 teaspoons fresh lemon juice

4 medium cloves garlic

DIPPING SAUCE*

1/2 cup soft tofu

1/2 cup low salt mayonnaise or Vegenaise (a vegan alternative)

2 1/2 tablespoons date sugar

1 tablespoon toasted sesame oil

1 tablespoon vegan Worcestershire sauce

1 tablespoon lemon juice

2 teaspoons *Dr. Fuhrman's VegiZest*

continued...

ARTICHOKES WITH DIPPING SAUCE *continued...*

DIRECTIONS

Cut about an inch off the top of each artichoke.

Pour an inch of water, fresh lemon juice, and garlic into a steamer pot. Place artichokes into steamer basket. Cover and steam for about 40 minutes until inside leaves can be pulled out easily.

While artichokes are steaming, make the sauce by blending dipping sauce ingredients together until smooth and creamy. Remove to a dipping bowl.

Drain steamed artichokes upside down on a paper towel.

Peel off artichokes, leaf by leaf, dipping the tip (the part that was attached to the heart of the choke) into the sauce. The soft undersides of the leaves can be eaten as well as the artichoke heart.

*Yields: 1 cup

One Serving Contains:
CALORIES 159.5; PROTEIN 4.9g; CARBOHYDRATE 24.9g; FAT 6.2g; SODIUM 174.4mg

Asian Vegetable Stir Fry

MANDI
24.5

Serves: 4 — Prep Time: 45 minutes

INGREDIENTS

1/2 cup brown rice, uncooked

14 ounces extra firm tofu, cubed (or 1 cup cooked beans)

1 teaspoon Bragg Liquid Aminos or low sodium soy sauce

1/2 teaspoon crushed red pepper flakes

2 tablespoons Spike seasoning or any other no salt seasoning

4 tablespoons unhulled sesame seeds

SAUCE

6 tablespoons apricot 100% fruit spread

4 tablespoons natural peanut butter, no salt, or raw cashew butter

2 tablespoons peeled and chopped ginger root

4 cloves garlic, chopped

4 teaspoons *Dr. Fuhrman's VegiZest*

1/3 cup water

4 tablespoons *Dr. Fuhrman's Black Fig Vinegar* or balsamic vinegar

1 teaspoon arrowroot powder

continued...

ASIAN VEGETABLE STIR FRY   *continued...*

VEGETABLES

> 1/8 cup water
>
> 1 medium onion, cut into wedges and separated into 1-inch strips
>
> 4 cups broccoli florets, small
>
> 2 medium carrots, cut diagonally into 1/3 inch slices
>
> 4 medium red bell peppers, cut in 1" squares
>
> 1 cup sugar snap peas or snow peas, strings removed
>
> 2 cups bok choy, cut in bite-sized pieces
>
> 3 cups shiitake, porcini or cremini mushrooms or a mixture, stems removed
>
> 16 ounces fresh organic spinach
>
> 1/2 cup raw cashew pieces, lightly toasted* (optional)
>
> 20 ounces romaine lettuce, shredded

DIRECTIONS

> Cook brown rice according to package directions.
>
> TOFU - Preheat oven to 350 degrees.
>
> Marinate tofu for 30 minutes in liquid aminos, some of the red pepper, and Spike. Toss marinated tofu with sesame seeds.
>
> Bake sesame coated tofu on nonstick baking pan in oven for 30-40 minutes until golden.
>
> SAUCE - Place sauce ingredients, along with rest of red pepper flakes, in a high powered blender and blend until smooth. Remove to a small bowl and set aside.

continued...

Asian Vegetable Stir Fry   *continued...*

VEGETABLES - In a large pan, saute onions, broccoli, carrots, red peppers, and snap peas in water over medium-high heat for 5 minutes. Toss while cooking, adding more water as necessary to keep from scorching.

After 5 minutes, add bok choy, and mushrooms and cover. Simmer until vegetables are just tender. Remove cover and cook off most water.

Add spinach and toss until wilted.

Add apricot sauce and stir until all vegetables are glazed and sauce is bubbly hot, about 1 minute.

Mix in cashews and baked tofu.

Serve over warmed shredded romaine lettuce, and 1/4 cup cooked plain brown rice, per person.

Lightly toast cashew pieces in a pan over medium heat for three minutes, shaking pan frequently.

One Serving Contains:
CALORIES 336.8; PROTEIN 15.0g; CARBOHYDRATE 51.2g; FAT 11.2g; SODIUM 172.5mg

THIS RECIPE LOOKS HARDER THAN IT IS. IT IS WELL WORTH THE TIME IT TAKES TO MAKE IT SINCE IT'S GOOD ENOUGH FOR COMPANY!

ASPARAGUS WITH BLACK FIG DRESSING

MANDI
8

Serves: 4 — Prep Time: 20 minutes

INGREDIENTS

1/3 cup *Dr. Fuhrman's Black Fig Vinegar*

1 tablespoon *Dr. Fuhrman's VegiZest* or other no salt seasoning

3 tablespoons water

1 tablespoon Dijon mustard

1 tablespoon chopped fresh marjoram or 1 teaspoon dried

1 teaspoon minced garlic

1 tablespoon almond butter

1 tablespoon ketchup, low sodium

2 pounds asparagus, tough ends trimmed
  then cut on diagonal into 2-inch pieces

1 small red bell pepper, very thinly sliced

1/2 cup pecans, toasted* and chopped (optional)

DIRECTIONS

Boil vinegar in heavy small saucepan over medium heat until reduced by half, about 3 minutes. Pour vinegar into large bowl.

Combine water with no salt seasoning. Whisk into vinegar, along with mustard, marjoram, garlic, almond butter and ketchup. Set dressing aside.

continued...

Asparagus
with Black Fig Dressing   *continued...*

Sauté asparagus in small amount of water, stirring over high heat for 3 minutes, then cover and steam for 1 minute. Remove to a bowl.

In same pan, sauté bell peppers in a small amount of water for 1 minute.

Add asparagus and bell peppers to dressing; toss to blend well.

Sprinkle with pecans if desired.

Lightly toast pecans in a 200 degree oven for 3 minutes.

One Serving Contains:
CALORIES 103.8; PROTEIN 6.5g; CARBOHYDRATE 13.9g; FAT 2.7g; SODIUM 107.7mg

BAKED GARLIC PITA CHIPS

MANDI
0.5

Serves: 4 — Prep Time: 8 minutes

INGREDIENTS

2 whole wheat pitas

olive oil cooking spray (optional)

garlic powder

DIRECTIONS

Preheat oven to 375 degrees.

Split each pita in half horizontally. Spray pita halves lightly with olive oil, if desired, and sprinkle with garlic powder.

Cut each half in half and then into four sections to form triangles.

Place on baking sheet and bake for 8 minutes or until lightly browned and crispy.

Serve with salsa or hummus.

One Serving Contains:
CALORIES 85.1; PROTEIN 3.1g; CARBOHYDRATE 17.6g; FAT 0.8g; SODIUM 170.2mg

Baked Potato Fries

Serves: 4 — Prep Time: 15 minutes

INGREDIENTS

2 pounds Yukon Gold potatoes or sweet potatoes

4 cloves fresh garlic, pressed or 2 tsp garlic powder

1 tablespoon olive oil

2 teaspoons onion powder

no salt herb seasoning

DIRECTIONS

Preheat oven to 350 degrees.

Peel potatoes if not organic and cut into strips.

Mix remaining ingredients and toss with potatoes.

Bake for 30 to 45 minutes or until lightly golden and tender.

One Serving Contains:
CALORIES 194.2; PROTEIN 4.1g; CARBOHYDRATE 37.4g; FAT 3.6g; SODIUM 14.7mg

BLACK BEAN LETTUCE BUNDLES

MANDI
7.5

Serves: 4 — Prep Time: 10 minutes

INGREDIENTS

2 cups cooked or canned black beans, no salt

1/2 large avocado, mashed

1/2 green bell pepper, chopped

3 scallions, chopped

1/3 cup chopped fresh cilantro, chopped

2 tablespoons lime juice

1 teaspoon cumin

1 clove garlic, minced

1/3 cup mild salsa, low sodium

8 large romaine lettuce leaves

DIRECTIONS

Mash beans and avocado together with fork.

Mix with all remaining ingredients except lettuce.

Place approximately 1/4 cup of filling in center of lettuce leaf and roll like a tortilla.

One Serving Contains:
CALORIES 186.8; PROTEIN 10g; CARBOHYDRATE 29.2g; FAT 4.6g; SODIUM 139.3mg

BRAISED BOK CHOY

Serves: 4 — Prep Time: 15 minutes

INGREDIENTS

8 baby bok choy or 3 regular bok choy

1 tablespoon Bragg Liquid Aminos or low sodium soy sauce

2 cups coarsely chopped shiitake mushrooms, optional

2 large cloves garlic, chopped, optional

1 tablespoon unhulled sesame seeds, lightly toasted*

DIRECTIONS

Cover bottom of large skillet with 1/2 inch water. Add bok choy (cut baby bok choy in half lengthwise or cut regular bok choy into chunks).

Drizzle with liquid aminos. Cover and cook on high heat until bok choy is tender, about 6 minutes.

Remove bok choy and if desired, add mushrooms and garlic to the liquid.

Simmer liquid until reduced to a glaze. Pour over bok choy. Top with toasted sesame seeds.

Lightly toast sesame seeds in a pan over medium heat for 3 minutes, shaking pan frequently.

One Serving Contains:
CALORIES 108.3; PROTEIN 11.8g; CARBOHYDRATE 16.5g; FAT 2.4g; SODIUM 244.7mg

BROCCOLI VINAIGRETTE

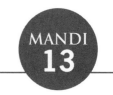

MANDI
13

Serves: 2 — Prep Time: 15 minutes

INGREDIENTS

1 large bunch broccoli

1/4 cup seasoned rice vinegar

1 tablespoon *Dr. Fuhrman's VegiZest*

2 teaspoons Dijon mustard

2 large cloves garlic, pressed or minced

DIRECTIONS

Chop broccoli into bite-sized florets. Peel stems and slice them into ¼ inch-thick strips.

Steam florets and stems for 8 minutes, or until just tender.

While the broccoli is steaming, whisk remaining ingredients in large bowl.

Add broccoli and toss to mix.

One Serving Contains:
CALORIES 110.7; PROTEIN 7.6g; CARBOHYDRATE 19g; FAT 0.9g; SODIUM 216.9mg

BROCCOLI WITH RED LENTIL SAUCE

**MANDI
17**

Serves: 4 — Prep Time: 15 minutes

INGREDIENTS

1/2 cup red lentils

1 medium onion, chopped

1 small clove garlic, chopped

1½ to 2 cups carrot juice

1 pound broccoli florets

1 tablespoon *Dr. Fuhrman's VegiZest*

1/2 teaspoon Mrs. Dash seasoning

1/2 teaspoon balsamic vinegar

1/4 cup chopped pecans (optional)

THIS DISH
FREEZES WELL.

DIRECTIONS

Add lentils, onions, garlic, and carrot juice to a saucepan. Bring to a boil, cover and simmer for 20-30 minutes until the lentils are soft and pale. Add more carrot juice if needed.

Meanwhile, steam the broccoli until just tender.

Put the cooked lentil mixture into a food processor or blender with the VegiZest, seasoning and balsamic vinegar and blend to a smooth puree. Add some carrot juice if it is too thick.

Place broccoli in a bowl and combine with sauce. If desired, top with chopped pecans.

One Serving Contains:
CALORIES 194.9; PROTEIN 11.7g; CARBOHYDRATE 38.7g; FAT 1.2g; SODIUM 83.4mg

BRUSSELS SPROUTS POLONAISE

MANDI
22

Serves: 3 — Prep Time: 10 minutes

INGREDIENTS

6 cups Brussels sprouts

1/4 cup soft tofu

2 tablespoons lemon juice

2 tablespoons date sugar

1 clove garlic, minced

1 tablespoon *Dr. Fuhrman's VegiZest*

1/2 cup chopped fresh parsley, chopped

1/2 cup soy milk

DIRECTIONS

Cut large sprouts in half. Steam for 8 minutes or until tender.

Blend tofu, lemon juice, date sugar, garlic, VegiZest, 1/4 cup parsley, and soy milk in blender and pour over sprouts.

Sprinkle with remaining parsley.

One Serving Contains:
CALORIES 139.5; PROTEIN 9.3g; CARBOHYDRATE 27.7g; FAT 1.6g; SODIUM 86.3mg

California Creamed Kale

MANDI
25

Serves: 4 — Prep Time: 10 minutes

INGREDIENTS

2 bunches kale,
leaves removed from tough stems and chopped

1 cup raw cashews

1 cup soy milk

4 tablespoons onion flakes

1 tablespoon *Dr. Fuhrman's VegiZest* (optional)

Sauce may be
used with
broccoli,
spinach, or
other steamed
vegetables.

DIRECTIONS

Place kale in a large steamer pot. Steam 10-20 minutes until soft.

Meanwhile, place remaining ingredients in a high-powered blender and blend until smooth.

Place kale in colander and press with a clean dish towel to remove some of the excess water. In a bowl, coarsely chop and mix kale with the cream sauce.

One Serving Contains:
CALORIES 268.8; PROTEIN 11.9g; CARBOHYDRATE 25g; FAT 15.9g; SODIUM 78.4mg

CAULIFLOWER, SPINACH MASHED "POTATOES"

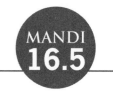

MANDI
16.5

Serves: 4 — Prep Time: 25 minutes

INGREDIENTS

6 cups cauliflower florets, fresh or frozen

6 cloves garlic, sliced

10 ounces fresh organic spinach or organic baby spinach

1/2 cup raw cashew butter

soy milk, if needed to thin

2 tablespoons *Dr. Fuhrman's VegiZest*, or to taste

1/4 teaspoon nutmeg

DIRECTIONS

Steam cauliflower and garlic about 8 to 10 minutes or until tender. Drain and press out as much water as possible in strainer.

Place spinach in steamer, steam until just wilted and set aside.

Process cauliflower, garlic, and cashew butter in a food processor with "S" blade in place until creamy and smooth. Check the consistency. If it is too thick, add a small amount of soy milk, process some more and check again.

Add VegiZest and nutmeg, adjusting to taste.

Mix pureed cauliflower with wilted spinach.

Serve hot or warm.

One Serving Contains:
CALORIES 166.6; PROTEIN 9.1g; CARBOHYDRATE 18.6g; FAT 8.5g; SODIUM 124.2mg

Chard and Vegetable Medley

Serves: 4 — Prep Time: 20 minutes

INGREDIENTS

1/2 cup water, divided

4 cloves garlic, minced or pressed

1 medium onion, coarsely chopped

2 tablespoons *Dr. Fuhrman's VegiZest*

1 teaspoon Spike no salt seasoning

4 small yellow squash, cut into 1/2 inch slices

2 bunches Swiss chard, red and green, coarsely chopped

1 large red bell pepper, cut into 1/2 inch slices

1 cup halved cherry tomatoes

2 tablespoons balsamic vinegar

DIRECTIONS

Place garlic, onion, VegiZest, Spike, and yellow squash in a large soup pot with 1/4 cup water. Bring to a high simmer. Cook until onion is soft, about 3 minutes.

Add remaining vegetables, along with another 1/4 cup water, and simmer covered for about 12 minutes or until tender. Drain vegetables, reserving liquid.

Add balsamic vinegar to liquid and reduce over high heat until syrupy.

Pour over vegetables.

One Serving Contains:
CALORIES 91.6; PROTEIN 5.8g; CARBOHYDRATE 19.8g; FAT 0.6g; SODIUM 184.1mg

CUBAN BLACK BEANS
WITH BROWN RICE

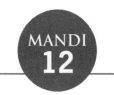

MANDI
12

Serves: 6 — Prep Time: 20 minutes

INGREDIENTS

4 cups brown rice, cooked

olive oil (small amount)

1 cup chopped onion

3/4 cup chopped green pepper

2 cups tomato juice, no salt

3 15-ounce cans black beans, (no or low salt) drained

1 14-ounce can whole tomatoes, (no salt) undrained and chopped

1 8-ounce can tomato sauce (no salt)

3 cloves garlic, minced

1 tablespoon *Dr. Fuhrman's VegiZest* or other no salt seasoning

1/2 teaspoon garlic powder

1/4 teaspoon black pepper

DIRECTIONS

Cook brown rice according to package directions.

Using a paper towel moistened with olive oil, lightly coat a large soup pot and sauté onion and peppers until tender.

Add tomato juice and next 7 ingredients; bring to a boil. Cover, reduce heat, and simmer 20 to 25 minutes or until vegetables are tender.

Serve with brown rice.

One Serving Contains:
CALORIES 489.5; PROTEIN 24.4g; CARBOHYDRATE 94.6g; FAT 2.9g; SODIUM 32.9mg

Eggplant Roulades

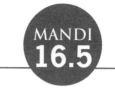

Serves: 6 — Prep Time: 25 minutes

INGREDIENTS

2 large eggplants,
   peeled and sliced 1/2" thick lengthwise

2 medium red bell peppers, coarsely chopped

1 medium onion, coarsely chopped

1 cup coarsely chopped carrots

1/2 cup chopped organic celery

4 cloves garlic, chopped

8 ounces organic baby spinach

1 tablespoon *Dr. Fuhrman's VegiZest* or other no salt seasoning

2 cups pasta sauce, no or low salt

6 ounces mozzarella cheese substitute, shredded

DIRECTIONS

Preheat oven to 350 degrees. Using a paper towel moistened with olive oil, lightly oil a non-stick baking pan. Arrange eggplant in a single layer. Bake about 20 minutes or until the eggplant is flexible enough to easily roll. Set aside.

In 1/8 cup water, sauté the bell peppers, onions, carrots, celery, and garlic until just tender, adding more water if needed. Add spinach and VegiZest. Transfer to a mixing bowl. Mix in 2 to 3 tablespoons of pasta sauce and shredded soy cheese.

In a baking pan, spread about 1/4 cup tomato sauce. Place some of the vegetable mixture on each eggplant slice, roll and place in baking pan on top of sauce.

Pour remaining tomato sauce over eggplant rolls. Bake 20 to 30 minutes or until heated through.

One Serving Contains:
CALORIES 186.6; PROTEIN 8.6g; CARBOHYDRATE 32.2g; FAT 4.3g; SODIUM 266.7mg

GARDEN STUFFED VEGETABLES

MANDI
21.5

Serves: 6 — Prep Time: 40 minutes

INGREDIENTS

2 medium zucchini

2 medium Portobello mushrooms

4 large peppers (use different colors for color vibrancy)

1/2 cup quinoa, rinsed well

1 small red pepper, chopped

1/2 pound shiitake mushrooms, chopped

3 whole green onions, chopped

2 stalks organic celery, chopped

1 stalk broccoli, chopped in small pieces

4 cloves garlic, chopped in small pieces

1 cup cooked lentils, or canned no or low salt, rinsed and drained

1/2 cup walnuts, coarsely chopped

2 ounces mozzarella cheese substitute, shredded

1/2 cup raisins

1/2 bunch parsley, chopped, divided

2 teaspoons Bragg Liquid Aminos or low sodium soy sauce

1 tablespoon *Dr. Fuhrman's VegiZest* or other no salt seasoning

2 cups pasta sauce, no or low salt

salad greens

1 tablespoon *Dr. Fuhrman's Black Fig Vinegar*
or balsamic vinegar, to taste

continued...

GARDEN STUFFED VEGETABLES   *continued...*

DIRECTIONS

Preheat oven to 350 degrees.

Prepare vegetables to be stuffed:

Trim off zucchini ends and cut in half lengthwise, scrape the seeds and some meat with a spoon, leaving the shell intact. Remove stems from the Portobello mushrooms. Slice off pepper tops and gently remove seeds.

On baking sheet, bake the zucchini and peppers for 5 minutes. Add mushrooms and bake for an additional 15 minutes.

Cook quinoa in 1 cup of water. Bring to a boil; turn down to low and simmer covered for 15 min. Take off heat and let it sit covered for 10 min.

In small amount of water, sauté red pepper, mushrooms, green onions, celery, broccoli and garlic until tender and water has cooked off.

In large bowl, mix cooked quinoa, lentils, walnuts, cheese substitute, raisins and 1/4 bunch chopped parsley with sautéed ingredients and season with liquid aminos and VegiZest.

Fill zucchini, mushrooms and peppers with quinoa mixture and place in a baking dish.

Spoon some pasta sauce over vegetables. Bake for 20-30 minutes until hot.

Serve on bed of salad greens which have been lightly tossed with *Dr. Fuhrman's Black Fig Vinegar* or balsamic vinegar.

Garnish vegetables with remaining chopped parsley.

One Serving Contains:
CALORIES 325.7; PROTEIN 14.4g; CARBOHYDRATE 51.7g; FAT 9.5g; SODIUM 217mg

HAWAIIAN SWEET POTATO PUDDING

MANDI
4.5

Serves: 4 — Prep Time: 15 minutes

INGREDIENTS

4 medium sweet potatoes (use organic for a sweeter taste)

1 cup orange juice

canned sliced pineapple (unsweetened), drained well

1 tablespoon date sugar (optional)

DIRECTIONS

Preheat oven to 400 degrees.

Prick sweet potatoes with a fork. Bake for 1 hour or until soft. Let cool and peel off skin.

Mash sweet potatoes in a food processor or high powered blender with orange juice and date sugar, if desired.

Spread mixture into a 9X9 inch glass baking dish. Cover with pineapple slices. Bake at 350 degrees for 1/2 hour.

One Serving Contains:
CALORIES 153.3; PROTEIN 2.6g; CARBOHYDRATE 36.1g; FAT 0.2g; SODIUM 72.3mg

LEMON ZEST SPINACH

MANDI
19

Serves: 4 — Prep Time: 10 minutes

INGREDIENTS
- 1 1/4 pounds fresh organic spinach or 4 bags organic baby spinach
- 6 cloves garlic, minced
- 5 tablespoons pine nuts
- 3 teaspoons lemon juice
- 1 teaspoon olive oil
- 1/2 teaspoon lemon zest

DIRECTIONS

Steam spinach and garlic until spinach is just wilted.

Place in bowl and toss in remaining ingredients.

One Serving Contains:
CALORIES 122.7; PROTEIN 5.8g; CARBOHYDRATE 8.4g; FAT 9.1g; SODIUM 113mg

MARIAN'S TOFU CHILI

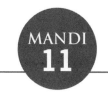

MANDI
11

Serves: 4 — Prep Time: 10 minutes

INGREDIENTS

3 cups cooked brown rice, optional

1 pound extra firm tofu, frozen and thawed*, squeezed dry and crumbled

1 medium green pepper, coarsely chopped

1/2 medium onion, coarsely chopped

2 cloves garlic, minced

1 28-ounce can chopped tomatoes, no salt

2 tablespoons chili powder, or more to taste

1/2 15-ounce can kidney beans (low or no salt), drained

1/2 15-ounce can pinto beans (low or no salt), drained

> IF DESIRED, THIS MAY BE MADE IN A CROCK POT. CRUMBLE FROZEN, THAWED TOFU INTO A LARGE PAN. TURN HEAT TO MED/HIGH AND ADD PEPPERS, ONIONS, AND GARLIC. COOK UNTIL TENDER. POUR INTO A CROCK POT ALONG WITH REMAINING INGREDIENTS. COVER AND COOK ON LOW FOR 6-8 HOURS OR ON HIGH FOR 3-4 HOURS.

DIRECTIONS

If using rice, cook according to package directions.

In a large pan, combine all ingredients except rice, and simmer for 30 minutes, or until all liquid is absorbed.

If desired, serve over brown rice.

*Thaw tofu on counter top for about 6 hours before squeezing out water. Freezing the tofu results in a more meaty texture. Unfrozen, crumbled tofu may also be used.

One Serving Contains:
CALORIES 298.2; PROTEIN 15.7g; CARBOHYDRATE 55.3g; FAT 3.6g; SODIUM 81.4mg

No Pasta Vegetable Lasagna

MANDI
26.5

Serves: 8 — Prep Time: 60 minutes

INGREDIENTS - LASAGNA "NOODLES"

2 large eggplants, sliced 1/4 inch lengthwise

3 small zucchini, slice lengthwise as thin as possible

3 small yellow squash, slice lengthwise as thin as possible

INGREDIENTS - TOFU RICOTTA"

1 package silken firm tofu

1 small onion, cut in quarters

4 cloves garlic, cut in half

1 bunch fresh basil leaves

1 1/4 pounds firm tofu

4 tablespoons *Dr. Fuhrman's VegiZest*

2 tablespoons dried Italian herbs

1 cup grated soy mozzarella cheese

INGREDIENTS - VEGETABLES

2 bunches broccoli florets & peeled stems, coarsely chopped

4 cups sliced mushrooms,
 (preferably a mixture of shiitake, cremini, oyster)

4 medium bell peppers (a mixture of red, yellow & orange), chopped

1 7-ounce bag organic baby spinach

3 cups pasta sauce, no or low salt

fresh basil, shredded

continued...

NO PASTA VEGETABLE LASAGNA *continued...*

DIRECTIONS

Preheat oven to 350 degrees.

Step 1: Lasagna "Noodles"

Bake eggplant, zucchini and squash slices for 10 minutes until flexible but not completely cooked.

Step 2: Tofu "Ricotta"

Puree soft tofu, onion, and garlic in a food processor. Add 1 bunch basil leaves and pulse to coarsely chop.

Squeeze firm tofu to remove excess water and crumble. Mix pureed soft tofu mixture with crumbled firm tofu. Add VegiZest, Italian herbs, and grated soy mozzarella cheese.

Step 3: Sauté Vegetables

Sauté broccoli, mushrooms, peppers, and spinach over low heat for 5 minutes, without water, just until tender.

Step 4: Assemble

Spread a thin layer of pasta sauce on bottom of a baking dish. Layer eggplant slices, then sautéed vegetables, tofu ricotta, squash and zucchini slices and spread with pasta sauce. Repeat layers ending with tofu ricotta. Spread pasta sauce on the top and bake, uncovered, for 1 hour or until hot and bubbly. Garnish with shredded fresh basil.

One Serving Contains:
CALORIES 277.6; PROTEIN 14.9g; CARBOHYDRATE 50.7g; FAT 4.9g; SODIUM 194mg

Orange Sesame Kale

MANDI
24

Serves: 4 — Prep Time: 15 minutes

INGREDIENTS

3/4 cup raw cashew butter or almond butter

2/3 cup orange juice

2 teaspoons *Dr. Fuhrman's VegiZest*

2 bunches kale, leaves removed from tough stems and chopped

2 tablespoons unhulled sesame seeds, lightly toasted*

DIRECTIONS

With a wire whisk, combine nut butter, orange juice, and VegiZest.

Steam kale for 15 to 20 minutes, turning halfway through cooking.

Combine steamed kale and cashew butter mixture.

Sprinkle with toasted sesame seeds.

*Lightly toast sesame seeds in a 200 degree oven for 3 minutes.

One Serving Contains:
CALORIES 343.2; PROTEIN 11.8g; CARBOHYDRATE 22g; FAT 26.1g; SODIUM 45.9mg

PASTA WITH ROASTED VEGETABLES

MANDI
8.5

Serves: 6 — Prep Time: 30 minutes

INGREDIENTS

2 red bell peppers, cut into 1/2 inch pieces

1 medium eggplant, unpeeled, cut into 1/2 inch pieces

1 large yellow crookneck squash, cut into 1/2 inch pieces

1 1/2 cups 1/2 inch pieces peeled butternut squash

2 tablespoons olive oil, divided

1 pound whole wheat or whole grain pasta

2 medium tomatoes, cored, seeded, diced

1/2 cup chopped fresh basil, chopped or 1 1/2 tablespoons dried

2 tablespoons balsamic vinegar or 1 tablespoon fresh lemon juice

2 cloves garlic, minced

DIRECTIONS

Preheat oven to 450 degrees.

Wipe large roasting pan with a thin coating of olive oil. Combine red bell peppers, eggplant, yellow squash, and butternut squash in prepared pan. Drizzle with 1 tablespoon olive oil and toss to coat.

Roast until vegetables are tender and beginning to brown, stirring occasionally, about 25 minutes.

Meanwhile, cook pasta and drain, reserving 1/2 cup cooking liquid.

Combine pasta, roasted vegetables, tomatoes, and basil in large bowl.

Add remaining tablespoon of oil, vinegar and garlic. Toss to combine.

Add cooking liquid by tablespoons to moisten, if desired.

One Serving Contains:
CALORIES 364.9; PROTEIN 14.4g; CARBOHYDRATE 71.5g; FAT 6g; SODIUM 13.7mg

Portobello - Red Pepper Sandwich

Serves: 4 — Prep Time: 25 minutes

INGREDIENTS - SANDWICH

1/2 large red onion, thinly sliced

4 large Portobello mushrooms, stems removed

4 (4 inch) whole wheat pitas

2 cups large arugula leaves

2 medium drained roasted red bell peppers, from jar, seeded and cut into 1/2-inch-thick slices

INGREDIENTS - TAHINI SPREAD

3/4 cup raw tahini (pureed sesame seeds)

1/2 cup water

1 tablespoon fresh lemon juice

1 tablespoon *Dr. Fuhrman's VegiZest*

1 teaspoon Bragg Liquid Aminos or low sodium soy sauce

1 large pitted medjool date, chopped or 2 deglet noor

1 small clove garlic, chopped

DIRECTIONS

Preheat oven to 375 degrees.

Arrange mushrooms and onions on baking sheet and roast until tender, about 15 to 20 minutes.

Meanwhile, make tahini spread by blending all spread ingredients together.

continued...

PORTOBELLO - RED PEPPER SANDWICH   *continued...*

When mushrooms/onions are done, split pitas in half horizontally and warm slightly. Spread generous amount of tahini spread on top half of split pita. Place 1/2 cup arugula on bottom half and then, 1 mushroom cap (pat dry with paper towels to absorb liquid), sliced onion and roasted red pepper.

One Serving Contains:
CALORIES 491.4; PROTEIN 17.5g; CARBOHYDRATE 61.7g; FAT 23.6g; SODIUM 456mg

QUICK VEGETABLE BEAN MEDLEY

MANDI
13

Serves: 4 — Prep Time: 15 minutes

INGREDIENTS

1 head broccoli, small florets, with peeled and sliced 1/2" thick stems

1 red bell pepper, thinly sliced

8 cloves garlic, chopped

1/2 pound shiitake mushrooms, sliced

2 15-ounce cans red beans, no salt, drained

1/3 cup water

1 tablespoon *Dr. Fuhrman's VegiZest*, or other no salt seasoning

1/3 cup sunflower seeds, lightly toasted

DIRECTIONS

In large pan, place all ingredients except the sunflower seeds. Sauté about 10 minutes or until broccoli is just tender. Toss in cooking juice and top with sunflower seeds.

One Serving Contains:
CALORIES 413.1; PROTEIN 27.5g; CARBOHYDRATE 64.9g; FAT 8.2g; SODIUM 55.8mg

RAISIN COLLARDS AND CARROTS

MANDI
31.5

Serves: 4 — Prep Time: 20 minutes

INGREDIENTS - VEGETABLES

4 bunches collard greens, leaves removed from tough stems and chopped

4 carrots, grated

INGREDIENTS - SAUCE

1 medium cucumber

1/2 cup raisins

1/4 cup raw almond butter

2 teaspoons *Dr. Fuhrman's Riesling Raisin Vinegar* (optional)

1 teaspoon nutritional yeast

1/2 cup currants (optional)

DIRECTIONS

Steam collard greens for 15 minutes. Add grated carrots and steam another 5 minutes.

Blend all sauce ingredients in a high powered blender until smooth. Add sauce to collards/carrots mixture and toss.

If desired, stir in currants.

One Serving Contains:
CALORIES 234.5; PROTEIN 7.6g; CARBOHYDRATE 34.6g; FAT 10.1g; SODIUM 76.5mg

ROASTED MIXED VEGETABLES

MANDI
18.5

Serves: 6 — Prep Time: 20 minutes

INGREDIENTS

3 cups brown rice (optional)

1 teaspoon olive oil or olive oil spray

1/2 pound Brussels sprouts

1 pound broccoli florets

1 pound cauliflower florets

1/2 pound baby carrots, cut in half

1/2 pound asparagus, hard ends removed and cut into 2" pieces

6 cloves garlic, minced

2 tablespoons *Dr. Fuhrman's Black Fig Vinegar*, or balsamic vinegar

2 teaspoons Bragg Liquid Aminos or low sodium soy sauce

> YOU MAY USE FROZEN VEGETABLES.

DIRECTIONS

Preheat oven to 450 degrees. If serving over rice, cook according to package directions.

To prepare Brussels sprouts, cut off stem base, peel outer leaves and cut a cross 1/4" deep in base of stem.

Lightly spray vegetables with olive oil and toss all ingredients, except rice, in a large bowl. Pour into a large baking pan and spread evenly.

Bake for 30 minutes, stirring after 15 minutes. If vegetables begin to get too brown before they are tender, pile them up to keep moist, turn heat down to 350 degrees and finish cooking.

Serve over brown rice, if desired.

One Serving Contains:
CALORIES 198.3; PROTEIN 8.8g; CARBOHYDRATE 40.8g; FAT 1.4g; SODIUM 165.8mg

ROASTED VEGETABLE PIZZA

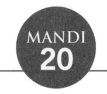

MANDI
20

Serves: 2 — Prep Time: 25 minutes

INGREDIENTS

2 cups broccoli florets

1 large red bell pepper, sliced 1 inch thick

1 large Portobello mushroom, sliced 1/2 inch thick

1 teaspoon garlic powder

1/2 teaspoon Bragg Liquid Aminos or low sodium soy sauce

1 tablespoon balsamic vinegar

1 teaspoon Mrs. Dash seasoning or Spike no salt seasoning

5 ounces organic baby spinach

2 whole grain tortillas

1/2 cup pasta sauce, no or low salt

2 ounces soy cheese or skim-milk cheese, grated

DIRECTIONS

Preheat oven to 350 degrees.

Toss broccoli, bell peppers, and mushrooms with garlic powder, liquid aminos, balsamic vinegar, and seasoning. Roast seasoned vegetables on a cookie sheet for 30 minutes, turning occasionally and mounding to keep from drying out.

Steam spinach until just wilted.

Remove vegetables when done and preheat oven to 450 degrees.

Spread a thin layer of pasta sauce on tortilla, sprinkle soy cheese, and distribute roasted vegetables and spinach on top.

Bake for approximately 7 minutes or until cheese is melted and tortilla is lightly brown around edges. Serve over brown rice, if desired.

One Serving Contains:
CALORIES 235.1; PROTEIN 13.5g; CARBOHYDRATE 35.8g; FAT 5.7g; SODIUM 362.9mg

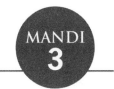

MANDI
3

SCRAMBLED TOFU

Serves: 2 — Prep Time: 10 minutes

INGREDIENTS

1 small onion (or several green onions), chopped

1/2 cup finely chopped green pepper

2 garlic cloves, chopped

2 cups drained and crumbled firm tofu

black pepper, Dr.Fuhrman's VegiZest, or Mrs. Dash seasoning, to taste

DIRECTIONS

In a large skillet, sauté onion, green pepper, and garlic in 1/4 cup water for 5 minutes.

Add the tofu and seasoning and cook for another 5 minutes.

One Serving Contains:
CALORIES 158.8; PROTEIN 5.8g; CARBOHYDRATE 30.5g; FAT 2.3g; SODIUM 25.8mg

SIMPLE BEAN BURGERS

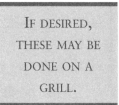

MANDI
3

Serves: 6 — Prep Time: 10 minutes

INGREDIENTS

1/4 cup sunflower seeds

2 cups canned red or pink beans, low or no salt, drained

1/2 cup minced onion

2 tablespoons ketchup, low sodium

1 tablespoon wheat germ or oats

1/2 teaspoon chili powder

> IF DESIRED,
> THESE MAY BE
> DONE ON A
> GRILL.

DIRECTIONS

Preheat oven to 350 degrees.

Chop the sunflower seeds in a food processor or hand chopper.

Mash the beans with a potato masher or food processor and mix with sunflower seed meal.

Mix in the remaining ingredients and form into six patties.

Lightly oil baking sheet with a little olive oil on a paper towel. Place patties on the pan and bake for 25 minutes.

Remove from the oven and let cool, about 10 minutes, until you can pick up each patty and compress it firmly in your hands to re-form the burger.

Turn patties over and bake another 10 minutes.

One Serving Contains:
CALORIES 126.7; PROTEIN 6.6g; CARBOHYDRATE 18.3g; FAT 3.6g; SODIUM 5.1mg

SOUTHWEST VEGETABLE CHILI

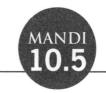

Serves: 3 — Prep Time: 20 minutes

INGREDIENTS

1 large potato, cut into small pieces

1 teaspoon olive oil

1/2 medium green bell pepper, chopped

1/2 medium red bell pepper, chopped

1/2 medium onion, chopped

1-2 small jalapeno peppers, seeded and chopped

2 large cloves garlic, chopped

1 1/2 tablespoons chili powder

1 14-ounce can chopped tomatoes

1 cup fresh or frozen corn

1 15-ounce can black beans (low or no salt), drained

2 tablespoons chopped fresh cilantro

> POTATO DOES NOT NEED TO BE PEELED IF ORGANIC.

DIRECTIONS

Place potatoes in a pot and cover with water. Simmer for about 8 minutes until tender. Drain and set aside.

Heat oil in a large saucepan over medium heat. Add green and red peppers, onions, jalapenos, and garlic and sauté for 2 minutes. Add chili powder and stir for one minute. Add tomatoes, corn, beans, cilantro, and reserved potatoes. Simmer until potatoes are very tender, stirring occasionally, for about 10 minutes.

One Serving Contains:
CALORIES 363.8; PROTEIN 17.7g; CARBOHYDRATE 70.8g; FAT 3.8g; SODIUM 71.3mg

SPAGHETTI SQUASH PRIMAVERA

MANDI
16.5

Serves: 4 — Prep Time: 20 minutes

INGREDIENTS

1 medium spaghetti squash

1 1/2 carrots, diagonally sliced

1/2 cup organic celery, diagonally sliced

3 cloves garlic, minced

1 1/2 cups shredded cabbage

1 small zucchini, chopped into small pieces

1 16-ounce can pinto beans, no or low salt, drained

1 14-ounce chopped tomatoes, no salt, drained

1/3 cup apple juice

1 teaspoon dried thyme

1 teaspoon dried parsley

1/2 teaspoon garlic powder

1 cup pasta sauce, no or low salt

1 head romaine lettuce leaves (optional)

DIRECTIONS

Preheat oven to 350 degrees.

Slice spaghetti squash in half lengthwise; remove seeds. Place both halves upside down on a baking sheet. Bake for 45 minutes.

Meanwhile, cook carrots and celery in 2 tablespoons of water in a covered pan over medium heat for 10 minutes, stirring occasionally.

continued...

Spaghetti Squash Primavera *continued...*

Add a little more water if needed. Add garlic, cabbage, and zucchini and cook, covered, for another 10 minutes. Stir in remaining ingredients, except for pasta sauce. Cover and simmer for 10 minutes or until carrots are tender.

When squash is done remove from oven and, using a fork, scrape spaghetti-like strands from squash into a bowl. Add pasta sauce and combine by mixing thoroughly.

Mix the vegetables, beans & herbs with the squash/pasta sauce mixture and serve on a bed of shredded romaine lettuce, if desired, or place back in the hollowed out squash bowls.

One Serving Contains:
CALORIES 289; PROTEIN 18.2g; CARBOHYDRATE 57.7g; FAT 1.9g; SODIUM 77.8mg

SPEEDY VEGETABLE WRAP

MANDI
10

Serves: 2 — Prep Time: 12 minutes

INGREDIENTS

2 whole wheat tortillas or whole wheat pitas

1 tablespoon fat free dressing, divided for1/2 tablespoon per wrap)

2 cups broccoli slaw mix

1 large tomato, diced

2 slices soy cheese or fat-free cheese, shredded

PREPACKAGED BROCCOLI SLAW CAN BE PURCHASED IN THE PRODUCE SECTION OF MANY MARKETS. COLE SLAW MIX, SHREDDED CABBAGE, OR SHREDDED BROCCOLI MAY ALSO BE USED.

DIRECTIONS

Spread fat free dressing over tortillas. Add broccoli slaw mix, tomatoes, and soy cheese.

Place in toaster oven or microwave just long enough to melt the cheese.

Roll up tortillas enclosing filling. If making pitas, stuff with dressing, vegetable, and cheese and serve without heating.

One Serving Contains:
CALORIES 262.9; PROTEIN 14.2g; CARBOHYDRATE 47.5g; FAT 4.5g; SODIUM 497.4mg

SPINACH AND BRUSSELS SPROUTS DELIGHT

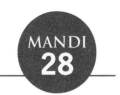

MANDI
28

Serves: 4 — Prep Time: 15 minutes

INGREDIENTS

16-ounces Brussels sprouts

14-ounces organic baby spinach

1/4 cup water

4 cloves garlic, minced

1 small onion, chopped

1 14.5-ounce can chopped tomatoes (no salt)

1 tablespoon *Dr. Fuhrman's VegiZest*

DIRECTIONS

Steam Brussels sprouts and spinach together for 8 minutes or until Brussels sprouts are almost tender.

Meanwhile, water sauté garlic and onion in a large pot until onions are tender, about 5 minutes. Add Brussels sprouts and spinach, along with chopped tomatoes and VegiZest. Simmer for an additional 10 minutes.

One Serving Contains:
CALORIES 109.9; PROTEIN 10.9g; CARBOHYDRATE 22.2g; FAT 1g; SODIUM 123.8mg

STEAMED BROCCOLI AND GARLIC

MANDI
12

Serves: 4 — Prep Time: 8 minutes

INGREDIENTS

2 pounds broccoli florets and peeled, chopped stems

6 cloves garlic, sliced

2 teaspoons olive oil

DIRECTIONS

Drizzle raw broccoli with 1 teaspoon olive oil and toss thoroughly. In steamer, cover and steam broccoli and garlic for 10 minutes.

Drizzle with remaining teaspoon of olive oil and toss.

One Serving Contains:
CALORIES 113.7; PROTEIN 6.7g; CARBOHYDRATE 16.5g; FAT 4.2g; SODIUM 75.7mg

THAI VEGETABLE CURRY

Serves: 8 — Prep Time: 40 minutes

INGREDIENTS

4 cups brown rice or quinoa, cooked

4 cloves garlic, finely chopped

2 tablespoons peeled and finely chopped fresh ginger

2 tablespoons chopped fresh mint

2 tablespoons chopped fresh basil

2 tablespoons chopped fresh cilantro

2 cups carrot juice

1 red bell pepper, thinly sliced

1 large eggplant, peeled, if desired & cut into 1 inch cubes

2 cups green beans, cut in 2 inch lengths

3 cups sliced shiitake mushrooms, stems removed

1 small can bamboo shoots

2 tablespoons *Dr. Fuhrman's VegiZest* or other no salt seasoning

1/2 teaspoon curry powder

3 tablespoons chunky peanut butter, natural unsalted

2 pounds tofu, cut into 1/4" thick slices

1/2 cup light coconut milk

2 cups watercress leaves, divided

1/2 cup chopped raw cashews

mint, basil, cilantro unchopped (for garnish, if desired)

continued...

THAI VEGETABLE CURRY   *continued...*

DIRECTIONS

Cook brown rice or quinoa according to package directions and set aside until ready to serve.

Add remaining ingredients (except for peanut butter, tofu, coconut milk, 1 cup of the watercress and cashews) to wok or large skillet. Bring to a boil and simmer covered, stirring occasionally, until all vegetables are tender. Mix in peanut butter. Add tofu, simmer and toss until hot.

Add coconut milk and heat through.

Serve on rice or quinoa. Top with the remaining cup of watercress and cashews.

One Serving Contains:
CALORIES 397.6; PROTEIN 13.5g; CARBOHYDRATE 60.9g; FAT 13.5g; SODIUM 51.2mg

FROZEN VEGETABLES MAY BE USED INSTEAD OF FRESH.

TUSCAN PASTA WITH TOMATOES AND ARUGULA

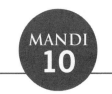

Serves: 4 — Prep Time: 15 minutes

INGREDIENTS

1 pound whole wheat fettuccine

1 tablespoon olive oil

1/4 teaspoon crushed red pepper

4 cloves garlic, thinly sliced

2 cups halved yellow cherry tomatoes

2 cups halved red cherry tomatoes

3 tablespoons lemon juice

10 ounces arugula

DIRECTIONS

Cook pasta according to package directions. Drain and retain 1 cup cooking liquid.

Meanwhile, heat oil in a large nonstick skillet over medium heat.

Add pepper and garlic to skillet; cook 1 minute or until garlic is fragrant. Add tomatoes, cook 1 minute or just until heated, stirring gently.

Remove skillet from heat, stir in lemon juice.

Combine hot pasta, arugula and warm tomato mixture in a large bowl, tossing to coat. If needed, add some of the cooking liquid from pasta to moisten.

One Serving Contains:
CALORIES 475.2; PROTEIN 20.1g; CARBOHYDRATE 95g; FAT 5.8g; SODIUM 49.1mg

VEGETABLE BURRITO

MANDI
5.5

Serves: 5 — Prep Time: 20 minutes

INGREDIENTS

1/2 tablespoon olive oil

1 medium onion, thinly sliced

1 medium red or green pepper, thinly sliced

1 medium zucchini, chopped

1/4 teaspoon chili powder

1 medium tomato, chopped

1 avocado, sliced

5 whole grain tortilla wraps

1 lime

DIRECTIONS

Saute onions, peppers, and zucchini in olive oil over med/high heat about 8 minutes until tender. Stir in chili powder.

Place sauteed vegetables, chopped tomatoes, and 2 slices of avocado on each tortilla.

Add squeeze of lime juice and roll up.

One Serving Contains:
CALORIES 227.2; PROTEIN 6.1g; CARBOHYDRATE 31.4g; FAT 10.2g; SODIUM 217.7mg

Vegetable Garbanzo Wrap

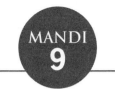

Serves: 4 — Prep Time: 20 minutes

INGREDIENTS

1 large tomato, chopped

1 avocado, chopped

1 cucumber, chopped

4 leaves romaine lettuce, shredded

1 15-ounce can garbanzo beans (low or no salt), drained and mashed

2 tablespoons fruit flavored vinegar

4 whole grain tortillas

1/2 tablespoon raw sesame tahini

DIRECTIONS

Toss vegetables with garbanzo beans and vinegar.

Warm a whole grain tortilla, spread a thin coating of tahini on it, and roll with the vegetable/bean mixture.

One Serving Contains:
CALORIES 555.8; PROTEIN 20.7g; CARBOHYDRATE 84.8g; FAT 16.9g; SODIUM 364.4mg

VEGETABLE SHEPHERD'S PIE

MANDI
9.5

Serves: 6 — Prep Time: 35 minutes

INGREDIENTS

4 large sweet potatoes

1 cup chopped broccoli

1 cup chopped cauliflower

1 medium leek, chopped

1 red bell pepper, cut into 1" squares

1 teaspoon herb de Provence
(dried French herbs)

4 tablespoons *Dr. Fuhrman's VegiZest*
or other no salt veggie soup base

2 cups chopped organic spinach, chopped

1/2 cup carrot juice

4 teaspoons cornstarch

1 cup firm tofu,
water squeezed out and crumbled

1 cup hazelnuts, brazil nuts, or almonds,
chopped medium fine (optional)

2 tablespoons chopped fresh parsley, for garnish (optional)

> FROZEN CHOPPED BROCCOLI, CAULIFLOWER AND SPINACH MAY BE SUBSTITUTED FOR FRESH. THAW AND DRAIN WELL. DO NOT PRE-COOK.

DIRECTIONS

Preheat oven to 375 degrees.

Bake sweet potatoes until soft, about 45 minutes. When potatoes are tender, remove to a bowl and mash.

continued...

VEGETABLE SHEPHERD'S PIE   *continued...*

Add broccoli, cauliflower, leeks, bell peppers, herb de Provence, and *Dr. Fuhrman's VegiZest* to a large sauté pan along with 2 cups of water. Simmer until almost tender (about 10 minutes). Add spinach and toss.

Drain vegetables, reserving vegetable liquid in pot.

Whisk cornstarch into carrot juice and whisk into boiling vegetable liquid until it thickens.

Add vegetables and crumbled tofu to sauce and toss to combine.

Divide mixture into two 8-inch pie pans. If desired, top with 1/2 cup nuts.

Spread sweet potatoes over the top and if desired, sprinkle with remaining nuts.

Bake at 375 degrees for 20-30 minutes until hot and hazelnuts are light brown. If desired, sprinkle with parsley.

One Serving Contains:
CALORIES 233.1; PROTEIN 7.2g; CARBOHYDRATE 34.8g; FAT 8.4g; SODIUM 104.5mg

THIS DISH MAY BE PREPARED AHEAD AND FROZEN, UNBAKED.
COVER TIGHTLY WITH ALUMINUM FOIL BEFORE FREEZING.
DO NOT DEFROST, BUT BAKE AN ADDITIONAL
10 TO 15 MINUTES.

VEGETABLES MILANESE

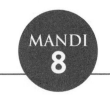

MANDI
8

Serves: 4 — Prep Time: 20 minutes

INGREDIENTS

1 head broccoli florets

2 cups baby carrots, cut into bite-sized pieces

1/2 head cauliflower florets

2 whole fennel bulbs, peeled and sliced

4 garlic cloves, pressed or minced

3 tablespoons *Dr. Fuhrman's Black Fig Vinegar*

2 teaspoons *Dr. Fuhrman's VegiZest*

2 teaspoons olive oil

1/3 cup pine nuts

1/4 cup chopped almonds, toasted*

1/4 cup fresh parsley, chopped

DIRECTIONS

Cover and steam broccoli, carrots, cauliflower, fennel and garlic for about 10 minutes. Do not overcook.

Whisk vinegar, VegiZest, and olive oil together. Drizzle over vegetables and toss with pine nuts.

Serve vegetables sprinkled with toasted almonds and fresh parsley.

Lightly toast almonds in a pan over low heat for 3 minutes, shaking pan frequently.

One Serving Contains:
CALORIES 269; PROTEIN 11.3g; CARBOHYDRATE 31.7g; FAT 14g; SODIUM 159.3mg

DESSERTS

APPLE SURPRISE

MANDI
5.5

Serves: 6 — Prep Time: 12 minutes

INGREDIENTS

1 cup raisins

1/4 cup water

8 apples, peeled, cored and diced

1/2 cup chopped walnuts

4 tablespoons ground flax seeds

1 tablespoon cinnamon

THIS RECIPE KEEPS
WELL IN THE
REFRIGERATOR FOR
SEVERAL DAYS.

DIRECTIONS

Place raisins in bottom of pot and cover with 1/4 cup water. Place diced apples on top. Cover and steam over very low heat for 7 minutes.

Transfer apple/raisin mixture to a bowl and mix well with remaining ingredients.

One Serving Contains:
CALORIES 259.6; PROTEIN 7.3g; CARBOHYDRATE 48.1g; FAT 8.8g; SODIUM 6.7mg

BANANA FIG ICE CREAM

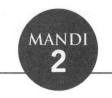

Serves: 4 — Prep Time: 6 minutes

INGREDIENTS

5 dried figs, stems removed

4 ripe bananas, frozen*

5 tablespoons soy milk

2 teaspoons *Dr. Fuhrman's Black Fig Vinegar*

DIRECTIONS

Blend all ingredients in a high powered blender until creamy.

Freeze ripe bananas at least 24 hrs in advance. To freeze bananas, peel, cut in thirds and wrap tightly in plastic wrap.

One Serving Contains:
CALORIES 176.2; PROTEIN 2.9g; CARBOHYDRATE 43.5g; FAT 1g; SODIUM 14.5mg

BANANA PUMPKIN PUDDING

MANDI
11.5

Serves: 2 — Prep Time: 10 minutes

INGREDIENTS

> 1/2 cup vanilla soy milk
>
> 5 dates, pitted
>
> 1 ripe banana, frozen*
>
> 1/2 15-ounce can pumpkin
>
> 2 ice cubes
>
> 1/4 teaspoon ground cinnamon
>
> 1/8 teaspoon ground mace or nutmeg

> STEAMED SQUASH
> COULD BE USED
> INSTEAD OF
> CANNED PUMPKIN.

DIRECTIONS

Place all ingredients in a high powered blender and process until smooth.

Spoon into custard cups. Chill at least two hours.

*Freeze ripe bananas at least 24 hrs in advance. To freeze bananas, peel, cut in thirds and wrap tightly in plastic wrap.

One Serving Contains:
CALORIES 179.8; PROTEIN 5g; CARBOHYDRATE 40.9g; FAT 1.8g; SODIUM 39.4mg

BANANA WALNUT ICE CREAM

MANDI
2.5

Serves: 2 — Prep Time: 2 minutes

INGREDIENTS

2 ripe bananas, frozen*

1/3 cup vanilla soy milk

1/2 ounce walnuts

DIRECTIONS

Blend all ingredients together in high powered blender until smooth and creamy.

*Freeze ripe bananas at least 24 hrs in advance. To freeze bananas, peel, cut in thirds and wrap tightly in plastic wrap.

One Serving Contains:
CALORIES 172.2; PROTEIN 4.2g; CARBOHYDRATE 29.9g; FAT 5.8g; SODIUM 23.3mg

BERRY COBBLER

MANDI
3.5

Serves: 2 — Prep Time: 2 minutes

INGREDIENTS

1 banana, sliced

1 cup frozen mixed berries

dash cinnamon

few drops vanilla extract

DIRECTIONS

Put banana into a small microwave safe bowl. Add frozen berries on top.

Sprinkle with cinnamon and add vanilla.

Microwave for about 3 minutes. Serve warm.

One Serving Contains:
CALORIES 78.6; PROTEIN 1g; CARBOHYDRATE 20.3g; FAT 0.3g; SODIUM 2.1mg

BLUEVADO PIE

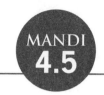

MANDI
4.5

Serves: 8 — Prep Time: 20 minutes

INGREDIENTS - CRUST

10 date/coconut rolls (remove almonds)

1 1/2 cups Familia, original swiss baby muesli, no added sugar (found in supermarkets)

INGREDIENTS - FILLING

10 ounces frozen blueberries

10 pitted dates, chopped

4-5 bananas

1 Haas avocado

1 teaspoon unsweetened shredded coconut

DIRECTIONS

For crust:

In a bowl, thoroughly blend the date/coconut rolls and muesli. Transfer mixture to pie plate, pressing down to make pie crust.

For filling:

In a high powered blender, blend all filling ingredients, except for coconut, until smooth.

Pour into the pie crust. Sprinkle with coconut.

Cover and freeze for at least 3 hours before serving.

One Serving Contains:
CALORIES 264.2; PROTEIN 4.3g; CARBOHYDRATE 53.2g; FAT 5.8g; SODIUM 13.6mg

FROZEN BANANA FLUFF

MANDI
2.5

Serves: 2 — Prep Time: 5 minutes

INGREDIENTS

1/4 cup vanilla soy milk

2 ripe bananas, frozen*

dash vanilla extract

2 tablespoons ground flax seeds (optional)

DIRECTIONS

Place the soy milk in the food processor, with the S blade in place (or use a high powered blender).

Turn the machine on and drop in small slices of the frozen bananas, one by one. Add vanilla and combine until smooth and creamy.

Sprinkle ground flaxseeds on top, if desired.

Freeze ripe bananas at least 24 hrs in advance. To freeze bananas, peel, cut in thirds and wrap tightly in plastic wrap.

One Serving Contains:
CALORIES 158; PROTEIN 3.9g; CARBOHYDRATE 30.5g; FAT 3.9g; SODIUM 19.8mg

FRUIT AND BERRY COMPOTE

MANDI
8.5

Serves: 4 — Prep Time: 10 minutes

INGREDIENTS

2 cups cubed fresh pineapple

1 cup halved organic strawberries

1 cup frozen cherries (pitted), thawed

1 cup dried fruit of choice, chopped (optional)

1/4 cup orange juice

2 oranges, peeled and cut into bite sized pieces

1 pear, peeled and cubed

1 tablespoon unsweetened shredded coconut (optional)

DIRECTIONS

Combine all ingredients except coconut.

Chill for two hours or refrigerate overnight.

If desired, sprinkle with coconut for garnish.

One Serving Contains:
CALORIES 241.8; PROTEIN 1.6g; CARBOHYDRATE 62.8g; FAT 0.6g; SODIUM 5.7mg

FRUIT AND NUT BOWL

MANDI
10

Serves: 2 — Prep Time: 10 minutes

INGREDIENTS

1 apple, cut into slices

1 banana, sliced

1 orange, sectioned

1/2 cup blueberries

1/2 cup sliced organic strawberries

2 tablespoons sliced raw almonds

2 tablespoons raw chopped walnuts

DIRECTIONS

Combine fruit and berries. Add nuts and toss gently.

One Serving Contains:
CALORIES 251.8; PROTEIN 6.2g; CARBOHYDRATE 41.5g; FAT 10g; SODIUM 4.7mg

HEALTHY CHOCOLATE CAKE

MANDI
9

Serves: 12   —   Prep Time: 40 minutes

INGREDIENTS - CAKE

1 2/3 cups whole wheat pastry flour

1 teaspoon baking powder

3 teaspoons baking soda

3 1/2 cups pitted dates, divided

1 cup pineapple chunks in own juice, drained

1 banana

1 cup unsweetened applesauce

1 cup shredded beets

3/4 cup shredded carrots

1/2 cup shredded zucchini

3 tablespoons *Dr. Fuhrman's Cocoa Powder*
  or other natural cocoa powder

1/2 cup currants

1 cup chopped walnuts

1 1/2 cups water

2 teaspoons vanilla extract

INGREDIENTS - CHOCOLATE NUT ICING

1 cup raw macadamia nuts or raw cashews, unsalted

1 cup vanilla soy milk

2/3 cup pitted dates

continued...

HEALTHY CHOCOLATE CAKE *continued...*

1/3 cup brazil nuts or hazelnuts

2 tablespoons cocoa powder

1 teaspoon vanilla extract

DIRECTIONS

Preheat oven to 350 degrees.

Mix flour, baking powder, and baking soda in a small bowl. Set aside.

In blender or food processor, puree 3 cups of the dates, pineapple, banana, and applesauce.

Slice remaining 1/2 cup dates into 1/2 inch thick pieces. In large bowl, mix sliced dates, beets, carrots, zucchini, cocoa powder, currants, walnuts, water, vanilla and flour mixture.

Add the blended mixture and mix well. Spread in a 9.5" X 13.5" nonstick baking pan.

Bake for 1 hour or until a toothpick inserted into the center comes out clean.

Icing:

Using a high powered blender*, combine all icing ingredients until smooth and creamy. Place a dollop over warm cake and serve. If desired, you may spread on cooled cake instead.

*A food processor may be used to combine icing ingredients but the icing will not be as smooth.

One Serving Contains:
CALORIES 454.1; PROTEIN 9.9g; CARBOHYDRATE 80.2g; FAT 15g; SODIUM 346.3mg

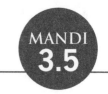

JENNA'S PEACH FREEZE

Serves: 2 — Prep Time: 8 minutes

INGREDIENTS

1 ripe banana, frozen

3 peaches or nectarines

2 medjool dates, or 4 deglet noor dates, pitted

1/4 cup vanilla soy milk

1 teaspoon vanilla

1/8 teaspoon cinnamon

DIRECTIONS

Cut up the banana and fruit.

Mix all ingredients together in a high powered blender.

One Serving Contains:
CALORIES 178.7; PROTEIN 3.9g; CARBOHYDRATE 41.8g; FAT 1.2g; SODIUM 17.6mg

MACADAMIA CREAM

MANDI
1.5

Serves: 8 — Prep Time: 5 minutes

INGREDIENTS

1 1/3 cups macadamia nuts

1 cup soy milk

2/3 cup dates, pitted

DIRECTIONS

Blend nuts, soy milk, and dates together in a high powered blender.

Serve over strawberries, other berries or fruit. May also be used as a topping on a fruit sorbet or fruit compote.

One Serving Contains:
CALORIES 217.8; PROTEIN 3.5g; CARBOHYDRATE 15.7g; FAT 17.6g; SODIUM 17.9mg

FOR A DIFFERENT FLAVOR, SUBSTITUTE DRIED MANGOS FOR HALF THE DATES. SOAK THE DRIED MANGOS IN THE SOY MILK OVERNIGHT.

MANGO RIESLING COMPOTE

**MANDI
4.5**

Serves: 6 — Prep Time: 8 minutes

INGREDIENTS

1 10-ounce bag frozen peaches,
    thawed and cut into small pieces

3 fresh ripe mangos, or frozen mangos,
    thawed and cut into small pieces

1 cup unsulfured dried apricots

1/2 cup raisins

1/2 cup soy milk or almond milk

1/4 cup *Dr. Fuhrman's Riesling Raisin Vinegar*

THIS RECIPE SHOULD
BE MADE ONE DAY
IN ADVANCE.

DIRECTIONS

Mix all ingredients together and refrigerate overnight in a closed
container.

One Serving Contains:
CALORIES 193.8; PROTEIN 2.8g; CARBOHYDRATE 48g; FAT 0.9g; SODIUM 19mg

FROZEN MANGOS
AND PEACHES ARE
EASIER TO CUT
WHEN PARTIALLY
THAWED RATHER
THAN THAWED
COMPLETELY.

MIXED BERRY FREEZE

MANDI
8.5

Serves: 2 — Prep Time: 10 minutes

INGREDIENTS

1/4 cup soy milk or almond milk

1/2 ripe banana, frozen*

1 10-ounce package of frozen mixed berries

2 tablespoons ground flax seeds

DIRECTIONS

Place the soy milk in a food processor, with the S blade in place (or use a high powered blender). Turn the machine on and drop in small slices of frozen banana, one by one.

Add the berries and mix.

Place in serving bowls and top with flax seeds.

Freeze ripe bananas at least 24 hours in advance. To freeze bananas, peel, cut in thirds, and wrap tightly in plastic wrap. The same recipe can also be made with other frozen fruit.

One Serving Contains:
CALORIES 140.2; PROTEIN 3.5g; CARBOHYDRATE 25.3g; FAT 4.2g; SODIUM 21mg

NUTRIENT-RICH CHOCOLATE PUDDING

MANDI 13

Serves: 6 — Prep Time: 45 minutes

INGREDIENTS

1/3 cup lentils, rinsed

1/2 bunch kale, de-stemmed and torn into bite-sized pieces

1 small butternut squash, cut into bite-sized pieces

1/2 small beet, peeled and quartered

1/2 cup broccoli florets

1 small zucchini, chopped

1 tablespoon *Dr. Fuhrman's VegiZest* or other no salt seasoning

1/4 cup raisins

1/4 cup chopped dates

1/4 cup raw cashews

15 dates, pitted

1 1/2 tablespoons cocoa powder, unsweetened,

1 teaspoon vanilla extract

1/3 cup soy milk

2.5 ounces organic baby spinach

1/2 tablespoon maple syrup (optional)

continued...

NUTRIENT-RICH CHOCOLATE PUDDING   *continued...*

DIRECTIONS

In a covered large pot, simmer the lentils, kale, butternut squash, beet, broccoli, zucchini, VegiZest or other seasoning, raisins and dates with 4 cups water for about 45 minutes until vegetables are very tender, stirring occasionally.

Separate beets and place in separate bowl.

With slotted spoon, remove 2 cups of the cooked vegetables. Place in high powered blender and blend until very smooth. Add remaining ingredients (except the beets) and blend to a smooth and creamy pudding consistency.

Add beets 1/4 at a time and blend until mixture reaches desired "chocolate" color.

Pour into custard cups and chill.

> THIS IS GREAT TOPPED WITH A DOLLOP OF THE MACADAMIA CREAM AND A STRAWBERRY ON TOP FOR GARNISH.

One Serving Contains:
CALORIES 244.9; PROTEIN 8.2g; CARBOHYDRATE 51.3g; FAT 3.5g; SODIUM 49.0mg

POACHED PEARS WITH RASPBERRY SAUCE

MANDI
4.5

Serves: 2 — Prep Time: 10 minutes

INGREDIENTS

2 pears

1 teaspoon lemon juice

2/3 cup frozen red raspberries, thawed

1 teaspoon date sugar or 1 medjool date, pitted

DIRECTIONS

Peel the pears and leave the stems attached. Drizzle with lemon juice.

Microwave for 4 minutes. Do not drain.

Blend raspberries and date sugar or dates in a high powered blender until smooth. Mix with cooking liquid.

Top pears with raspberry sauce.

One Serving Contains:
CALORIES 151.5; PROTEIN 1.3g; CARBOHYDRATE 39.8g; FAT 0.5g; SODIUM 2.2mg

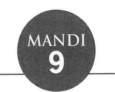

Strawberry Pineapple Sorbet

Serves: 2 — Prep Time: 5 minutes

INGREDIENTS

    1 10-ounce bag frozen strawberries

    1/2 cup orange juice or soy milk

    4 slices dried pineapple, unsweetened and unsulphured

    3 pitted dates

    1 cup fresh organic strawberries, sliced

DIRECTIONS

Blend all ingredients except fresh strawberries in a high powered blender.

Pour into sorbet glasses and top with sliced fresh strawberries.

One Serving Contains:
CALORIES 152.1; PROTEIN 1.8g; CARBOHYDRATE 38.6g; FAT 0.5g; SODIUM 6.9mg

VERY BERRY ICE CREAM

MANDI
6.5

Serves: 3 — Prep Time: 2 minutes

INGREDIENTS

1/2 package frozen organic peaches

1/2 package frozen organic mixed berries

1 cup apple juice

1 banana

DIRECTIONS

Blend all ingredients in in a high powered blender until smooth and creamy.

One Serving Contains:
CALORIES 129.8; PROTEIN 1.6g; CARBOHYDRATE 32.8g; FAT 0.5g; SODIUM 4.4mg

WILD APPLE CRUNCH

MANDI
3.5

Serves: 8 — Prep Time: 15 minutes

INGREDIENTS

6 apples, peeled and sliced

3/4 cup chopped walnuts

8 dates, chopped

1 cup currants or raisins

3/4 cup water

1/2 teaspoon cinnamon

1/4 teaspoon nutmeg

juice of 1 orange

> YOU CAN ALSO SIMMER THIS IN A COVERED POT FOR 30 MINUTES ON TOP OF THE STOVE, STIRRING OCCASIONALLY.

DIRECTIONS

Preheat oven to 375 degrees.

Combine all ingredients except the orange juice. Place in a baking pan and drizzle the orange juice on top.

Cover and bake at 375 degrees for about one hour until all ingredients are soft, stirring occasionally.

One Serving Contains:
CALORIES 207.4; PROTEIN 4.7g; CARBOHYDRATE 37.3g; FAT 7.5g; SODIUM 4.2mg

YUMMY BANANA-OAT BARS

MANDI
2.5

Serves: 8 — Prep Time: 10 minutes

INGREDIENTS

2 cups quick old fashioned oats (not instant)

1/2 cup shredded coconut

1/2 cup raisins or chopped dates

1/4 cup chopped walnuts

2 large ripe bananas, mashed

1/4 cup unsweetened applesauce (optional)

1 tablespoon date sugar (optional)

> ADD THE APPLESAUCE AND DATE SUGAR FOR A SWEETER, MOISTER VERSION OF THESE BARS.

DIRECTIONS

Preheat oven to 350 degrees.

Mix ingredients together in a large bowl.

Press dough in a 9"X 9" baking pan and bake for 30 minutes.

Cool on wire rack. When cool, slice into squares or bars and serve.

One Serving Contains:
CALORIES 250; PROTEIN 7.7g; CARBOHYDRATE 41.9g; FAT 6.9g; SODIUM 3.3mg

"Remember ... the prescription is nutrition."

~ JOEL FUHRMAN, M.D.

For more recipes and support visit
www.DrFuhrman.com